Annette Koshti-Richman

'THE UNOFFICIAL SELF-CARE GUIDE FOR CARERS'

A mother's journey transitioning the *tangled cobwebs* of children's to adults' services whilst sharing self-care tips

First published in Great Britain as a softback original in 2020

Copyright © Annette Koshti-Richman

The moral right of this author has been asserted.

All rights reserved.

No part of this publication may be reproduced, stored in a retrieval system, or transmitted, in any form or by any means, without the prior permission in writing of the publisher, nor be otherwise circulated in any form of binding or cover other than that in which it is published and without a similar condition including this condition being imposed on the subsequent purchaser.

Typeset in Sabon LT Std

Editing, design, typesetting and publishing by UK Book Publishing

www.ukbookpublishing.com

ISBN: 978-1-913179-99-1

In memory of my Godmother 'Aunty Dorothy' who was my inspiration to be a nurse, kept me sane during the dark days and will be forever in my heart.

'THE UNOFFICIAL SELF-CARE GUIDE FOR CARERS'

Mother's day wishes 2019!

Another mother's day is here
I'm getting more like you every year
My hair is now rather grey
My teeth more crowns than decay

I am now gardening at a slower pace
Slathering anti-wrinkle cream on my face
Only now it's my children's lives I'm tending
As happy mother's days wishes I am sending!

I had wrongly hoped that my life/our life would improve once Hedge reached 18 years of age. How wrong could I be? The so-called transition that started at the age of 16 continues to cause stress, anxiety and worry. As for me my light at the end of the tunnel for almost getting my career off the ground had also gone pear shaped in more ways than one and all due to the horrendous situation we all found ourselves in! Spin, spin and more spin and not a lot I could do to prevent further spin other than keep emailing, phoning and championing Hedge's corner. I continue to be weary from the previous 18 years of challenging and fear the worst.

Roll back to my previous book 'Tangled Cobwebs', where the services were a tangle of webs so tightly interwoven that it was a constant struggle to get Hedge the care and support he needed and yes life I suppose has changed. Hedge is now almost 21 years old and has still not transitioned to any adult mental health service. I have been forced into the situation of seeking alternative employment (having been in my previous job for only a year) and I continually try to keep my head above the bubbling vat of nothingness. I repeatedly question whether it is really possible to attempt self-care when it is difficult to even find time to boil an egg.

Early intervention and provision of mental health support could have prevented so much that we are now left dealing with as a family.

I ask myself "where did it all go so badly wrong?" ... well ...

CONTENTS

Why bother with Self-Care? 1
Writing down your cares away 3
Transition meetings 6
Transitions assessment 10
Imagine 14
Failed care packages 18
   Light at the end of the tunnel 20
   Christmas and Round Robins 25
The chance for a new career 28
Continuing issues at work 32
Here we go again 39
   Anxiety and its consequences 40
The curious case of being Hedge 43
   Time 46
Thinking of others before myself 48
Self-care Support Groups 52
   Give me a moment please 53
Friends and the great escape 58
Guinea pig trials 65
A child's answers to our prayers 72
Planning for the future 75
Self-care whilst gardening 80

Brexit	86
College dreams and losses	89
Being an appointee to Personal Independence Payments (PIPs)	93
Mug embossed across my forehead	99
Technology and self-care	103
Sleep	107
Computer use	111
Dearest 'The Hedge'	112
Bargain hunting	115
Embarrassing moments whilst attempting self-care	119
A day off to attempt self-care	122
A day to myself	126
Fruity frustrations	129
Out of the blue	133
Eccles cakes and friendship	139
A self-enforced break away	142
Returning from a few days' self-enforced break	145
Seeing things as they are	153
Toilet humour and self-care	156
Fabrications and little lies	160
Mother's Day with the Brownies	163
Decluttering for self-care	166
The tragic case of mistaken communication	169
Rising early to attempt self-care	173
Starting a new course	177
The tale of two kittens (who are utterly adorable)	181
Eating healthily (finally) to lose weight	187

Passing the hot potato	191
Seeing into the future	196
Juggling my life away	201
The spring of my winter	205
The storm after the calm	209
Finally taking stock of the situation	212
Then there was Covid-19	216
Wearing the dreaded face masks –– keep smiling	221
Lemons are great to suck on	225
It's an age thing	227
A final update	229
Acknowledgements	233

Why bother with Self-Care?

Self-care is something a lot of people are talking about these days. Note the lovely book cover that represents the web on the front cover of my previous book, well even this book cover demonstrates self-care. If you let your younger or older child push the wheelchair it can make them feel important and it allows you to amble along behind whilst eating sneaky sweets that you have stashed in your pocket. I am all for making children feel self-worth and importance!

With all the talk about self-care I guessed I might as well use the topic to my advantage and get on the band wagon. Mental health is gaining more publicity and there is priority by the Government and services (albeit from where I view it rather superficial), yet who is actually providing self-care or mental health support to carers? No-one teaches you to be a carer and no-one tells you how important it is to look after your own self-care. In actual fact they do, but it can be rather piecemeal and just a tick box exercise. No-one tells you the battles you will have whilst caring or the guilt you will feel, unless they are also a carer. I heard a lot about transition to adult services when Hedge was a child. Transition used to feel so far away and I had thought things would get easier. In some ways it has, as Hedge is an adult now and I can be blunter with people who try to accuse me of neglecting him as he is no longer my legal responsibility. Then in another way I see it as a load more challenging as Hedge is now expected to conform to the world as he continues not to fit the boxes that the health professionals expect him to fit in. Remember one thing and that is the fact that you matter and unless you take time for self-care you will end up more exhausted than you ever expected was possible. You count, and if it means taking a little bit of 'me time,' then you deserve it! The rest of the so-called world of support can go shove it somewhere less than desirable for the day and you can take a few moments for yourself, or at least try to!

Writing down your cares away

I have always loved writing and was first introduced to this when my grandmother gave me an old unused green leather diary. From the day she handed it to me I diligently kept a note of what had happened on that day (even if the dates didn't quite match as the diary was several years out of date). Some of my writings were typical of those of a young child and as I grew older it almost became a compulsion to write down everything that had happened and I would worry if I was a week behind in my writings. It was the deterioration in Hedge's health that permanently put the writings in my diary (or journal as it is now called), to a halt. I was far too busy juggling Hedge's ever-increasing health needs and appointments and the added anxiety it was causing me put an end to this life-long habit of mine. I am so grateful that I stopped as it has enabled me to channel my energy into something far greater, which was having my first book Tangled Cobwebs published and now writing my second.

My writings have helped to comfort and inform in other ways too as I have written in nursing journals regarding the effects of caring, amongst a whole host of other issues. I also post tips on Facebook that I have come across in my caring role. The one thing I never do in my writings is to criticise other care givers for what they are trying to do. I might be a tad sarcastic whilst I articulate about the care provided by services but I would never say anything online or anywhere else that I would not mind repeating. Hedge has always given his full consent to everything I have written and when he was a child I was always careful that what I wrote about him would not cause embarrassment later on in his life. Writings on the internet leave a footprint hence I have a fake Facebook name so that future employers or patients can't find me. I will never again write in a diary (or journal), but I will continue in my writings and campaigning for better services for everyone. Writing can help me express emotions, thoughts and dreams and let the creative side of me flourish.

> Writing down your cares away
> A great source of self-care
> Let your cares be written
> So on your sleeves you wear
>
> By writing down and expressing
> Thoughts and dreams appear
> Enabling stresses of the caring role
> To ease and disappear

If just for a moment or an hour
You can dissipate your woes
Once worries are written down
Your highs will surpass your lows

Self-care in the written form
A string of words outpoured
Memories and wishes transcribed
Your wellbeing safely restored

I am not in any way advocating anyone taking up or stopping writing in their journals as for many this will help. Purely highlighting the fact that if this activity is causing more grief than enjoyment, then think carefully like I did as to whether it is worth doing it at all. In my case I am grateful some days that I gave up writing in a journal; on other days it would have come in very handy as evidence for when I am endeavouring to demonstrate just how many times I have had to chase and chase again for someone to get back to me. Either embrace the inner author in you or simply don't bother otherwise it will become yet another chore on your list of ever-growing chores to do.

Transition meetings

"Oh my goodness," said with a sigh. We started the process with a whole day meeting in order to collectively piece together everything of the last 16 years. This was planned to ensure a smooth transition. Goodness knows what happens when there is no plan for a smooth transition as Hedge's transition has been one that I would not wish on my worst enemy. The report that was issued following the whole day meeting (over 30 pages long) was mainly ignored by the professionals. However, it did and continues to help when new carers need training as reading this report helps bring them quickly up to speed on what has led to Hedge's current issues. We have now had many more meetings that equate to over 100 hours of our time. It really is no wonder that services are stretched to breaking point when most of the time is spent in meetings, procrastinating about the same old issues yet again. Hedge prefers us to attend many of the meetings for him as he finds the whole process intimidating and stressful. Unsurprisingly we do too, but have to attend if we are to try to secure a future for Hedge.

Transition to adult services
A real eye opener indeed

TRANSITION MEETINGS

A united front meeting as one
Sounds better said than done

The meetings and the talking
The stress constantly increasing
The actions just kept growing
And paperwork steadily flowing

A simple process we were told
To help appreciate his needs
Allows his voice to shine through
And informs what he wants to do

So we patiently attended
Meeting after meeting
New professionals to reassess
Our lives on hold, a tangled mess

Politely accepting in good faith
More panels to be passed
And paperwork to complete
Our patience growing deplete

Oddly enough our child's needs
Change the second he turns 18
His care is now in adult services hands
And he doesn't quite fit the bands
(bands predetermine who funds for support)

'THE UNOFFICIAL SELF-CARE GUIDE FOR CARERS'

He's too good for one
Not bad enough for another
No pathway can be found
Caught in a care merry-go-round

One minute after midnight
A miracle has occurred
Doomed by a fundamental flaw
Hedge's needs are suddenly no more

Being sarcastic we wish we'd known
We wouldn't have stressed so much
We could've not bothered all those years
'cause at 18 any additional need disappears!

Only for us Hedge's needs continue to grow
His body fails to rejuvenate
His poor health doesn't go away
Nothing has changed since yesterday

However, I've just two simple questions
Who guides him when he's sick?
Who provides therapy or support?
I need time to digest and retort

Summing up it appears
Is it basically left all down to me

Hedge's needs are now forgot
Whilst services play pretend and sugar coat his lot!

After each meeting we attend we make sure that we do something positive on the way home, either a short drive to debrief over the view of the sea or if it was a particularly draining meeting we treat ourselves to a takeaway. Yet again we somehow squeeze in self-care where we can. Chips can be quite cheap and don't exactly break the bank and what better way of relaxing then burning your fingers as you try to pick up and eat a hot chip soaked in vinegar with a light sprinkling of salt? I can almost feel the stress easing away as my tastebuds come alive to the memory of chips. Ok so my car does stink afterwards and Little sis asks why the car is so smelly the next day on the school run and then accuses me of being greedy when she spies a dropped chip that has somehow missed my mouth the day before. However, it is these small things in life that come in the shape of chips that get me through the tough times. All wrapped up as a parcel of chips in the guise of self-care. What more could I or anyone else desire –– provided you like chips.

Transitions assessment

Andrew and I were obviously in complete denial when we attended the transitions meetings and assumed that this would equate to things going smoothly. After a battle between services it was decided that in order to 'give Hedge a voice and to let him flourish', Hedge needed to be assessed by an independent team of carers. Initially the local authority were prepared to spend something in the region of £750.00 a week on the accommodation alone for Hedge to reside in a care bungalow that he could 'flourish' in, whilst further funding to have the ratio of 2:1 staff (at an added cost) to assess what he could and couldn't do. We argued our point that this would prove very traumatising for Hedge and also questioned what would happen to the rest of his care team whom I employed through using a Personal Health Budget. Therefore it was conclusively agreed, after many lengthy negotiations, that Hedge could be assessed in our own home. An agency was chosen by the local authority after Hedge's profile had gone to brokerage. Eventually the agency came on board in order to assess Hedge's care needs, whilst also keeping on his current staff team that I employed. Talk about costly. Don't even start me on that one, as I dread to think how many other families are also going through the same ridiculous assessment process whilst wasting taxpayer's money. Then there was the small detail that left us reeling and this was how this could only happen if Andrew, Little sis and myself moved out! Great, so my disabled son, who has anxiety and mental health issues, can be at home whilst being assessed, but we couldn't be there at the same time as we might have influenced the assessment. The rationale for the entire process still leaves me deliberating how we got to the situation we did.

The next quandary was where exactly where we going to live. We contemplated staying on a local campsite for a few months (we were told it would take three months for the teams to properly assess Hedge's needs), but somehow visions of me being cooped up on a campsite trying to cook, wash and clean for three months didn't fill me with joy. We did look at one local campsite out of desperation but couldn't escape quickly enough when we drove up to the caravans to see that they were mainly workmen's caravans probably from local building sites who were using old caravans that had stood there for some time, as they were covered with a mossy green coating and a thick layer of grime. The portable toilets were equally unappealing and the happy campers were sat outside their caravans still sporting their high visibility clothes whilst downing bottles of larger.

Our next plan was to think about Andrew asking his mother if he could stay there and I would have to ask my parents if Little sis and I could move in with them. This was thought about and discarded quickly as thoughts of us splitting the family up even more was not something that we wished to do. We also had the small finer detail of having to get Little sis to and from school. We therefore spoke to my niece, who was renting the house we had built for Hedge, to explain the situation. The whole discussion made us feel dreadful and we even explored the option of them partially using our house next door where Hedge was to be assessed. The conclusion to this horrible episode was that my niece and her then partner (now husband) moved out and we moved in.

Only, as you and I know, you can't just move into an empty house, you need certain items, like beds, bedding, towels. So yet another stress for us as we were forced to buy two single beds, manhandle one of our sofas across our back garden into the new build and buy a cheap TV, get a chest of drawers and second-hand table and chairs. This was all whilst working and attempting to keep sane and care for Little sis and continually support Hedge's care needs.

I felt dreadful about my niece as it was just a few months before her wedding and something she could have justifiably done without. Being blunt, it was something we could all have done without. The resultant assessment left Hedge feeling spied upon. Most exasperatingly the results of the assessment provided the same conclusion as we told them it would. Hedge's care needs were to be fully health funded. It had cost us more than just a decision, it had cost us loads in emotional stress, made Hedge deteriorate in his mental health and left us feeling at an all-time low and shattered by how crazy the system is when trying to negotiate and get the care you need. Is this honestly how the government wants local authorities to behave towards families who are trying to get the care they need for their loved ones?

My self-care consisted of playing draughts with Andrew in the evenings due to the TV signal being so poor and getting to bed early as there was nothing to do in the evening. We also had lots of take-aways to eat as we hadn't had time or the funds to buy a fridge or freezer. Thankfully, as you already know, I adore chips. So yet again boredom and food in the shape of a good fatty chip helped save the day. Please note that I am ignoring the possibility of having high cholesterol or the fact that being a nurse I should be advocating a healthy diet. Somehow munching on salad leaves does not quite have the same effect as I am not a rabbit and it is far easier to eat chips than prepare a more wholesome salad. Although I do agree that a wholesome salad is less likely to keep me up with indigestion all night long due to eating chips so late in the evening.

(Hedge has now successfully moved into his new home, but as always nothing ever goes smoothly.)

Imagine

Imagine a world that really cares
A world that wants to improve
A world that doesn't make excuses
A world where mountains can move

A world without the stress
A world without all the worry
A world when all the professionals
Weren't continuously in a hurry

A world where money didn't matter
A world where funding was there
A world where parents/carers could sleep
Knowing that others do care

A world that didn't neglect
A world that turned a blind eye
A world that just accepted
And didn't keep questioning why

A world that recognised difference
A world that wanted all to achieve

IMAGINE

A world not requiring supporting evidence
But one that had the ability to believe

A world that was equal and fair
A world that didn't need campaigns
A world that just accepted
Not requiring messages on buses and trains

A world where difference is embraced
A world that recognised need
A world that treated everyone equally
And that therapy was given with speed

A world where families are recognised
A world that isn't budget led
A world understanding early intervention
Ends up saving money instead

A world that doesn't fob off
A world that isn't ring fenced so tight
A world that funding can move
So quality of life is a right

Sadly my world doesn't include me
Sadly my world is ignored and shattered
Sadly after years of caring for free
My dreams and hopes are battered

I don't even get the minimum wage
I don't qualify for any support
I don't even get acknowledged
Other than being mother in a report

I work 24 hours 52 weeks of the year
I receive no break in my quest
Employees have minimum break times
I don't even get five minutes' rest

I am a mother, wife and carer
I am a campaigner and appointment maker
A wheelchair pusher, a therapist
I am a mover and shaker

But it achieves precious little for me
I am now well past my best
I haven't even had a social life
Whilst I've been put to the test

The Government apparently thanks me
For saving them time and money
So whilst I am a carer
Why's my life far from sunny?

As I see no thanks other than wrinkles
I never see help coming my way

I never see support other than piecemeal
I am on house arrest, no choice but to stay

So thank you for forgetting me
Thank you for ignoring my health
Thank you for my zero salary
For helping prop budgets by stealth!

Failed care packages

It appears that I am to blame for the failed care package. After the lengthy process of assessments to fight it out between who would fund Hedge's care, it was no surprise that it was overwhelmingly agreed that Hedge would have 24/7 continuing healthcare funded by the NHS. Sadly my plea for extra hours to help me run Hedge's Personal Health Budget and a team of seven staff fell on deaf ears and we were told a firm 'No'. This created a huge amount of work for me as I was having to manage seven staff, their payroll, training, employment, recruitment, retention, meetings etc, not to mention managing the stock checking, ordering, risk assessments, care plans, insurances etc. I was left having to do these activities in the early hours of the morning or very late at night which ran into the early hours of the morning. Working my 32.5 hours and caring for Little sis, enabled me the escape I needed. Regrettably the lack of mental health support for Hedge and the Teflon shoulders of the teams turning him down for care, left me with rather a large problem. The problem was recruitment and retention of staff. I seemed to have no problem recruiting, spent hours of my time training, only for them to leave shortly afterwards due to not being able to cope or manage the mental health problems that Hedge exhibited and continues to have due to his Post Traumatic Stress Disorder and depression. Let me not pretend that recruiting staff was easy as that would be a lie. Recruiting staff meant me creating an advert on the Indeed Job site, asking potential candidates to phone me, compiling their details, emailing out applications forms, going through completed application forms, inviting to interview, interviewing, arranging for references checks, DBS (enhanced disclosure and barring service), booking training and also delivering training and arranging for shadow shifts. The most important bit was ensuring that there was a meet and greet that included Hedge so he also had the final say. Sadly some meets and greets ended up in a 'No' from Hedge and it was straight back to the drawing board again.

'On my knees' is one way of describing the process. At the front of my mind was the knowledge that one wrong decision on who to recruit could create an avalanche of issues for the rest of the staff team and give rise to others wishing to leave. I also had the joy of dealing with the complaints that came in from those who were leaving and having to manage many stressful situations that were not of my own making. I constantly explained to those I employed that an Insurance Company helped me manage my Human Resource (HR) issues, but that always seemed to fall on deaf ears. Within only one year I had one employee leave and take me to an employment hearing and the other leave and his angry wife scream and shout at me down the telephone to the point where I was left shaking on the other end of the receiver and emotionally shocked at what she was screaming at me. Being an employer, I was unable to say anything other than remain calm, otherwise I could have had anything I said used against me.

In total I consumed roughly five years of my life chasing for support for the care team by way of training for mental health and breakaway etc. This time and energy was eating away at my family time and I did my best to keep on top of everything but was beaten after the screaming wife of an employee verbally threatened me. It was the kick I needed and she did me a favour as I reflected and decided I had done enough to manage the Direct Payments via a Personal Health Budget and emailed the necessary people to tell them that I needed the help of an agency to support in the recruitment and employment of staff for Hedge.

Clearly I thought the process of using a care agency to provide care staff would have helped me out more than it did, otherwise I would have thought harder about making the decision. But in my mind there was no going back… Could there really be light at the end of the tunnel??

Light at the end of the tunnel

Light at the end of the tunnel
Can come quicker than you think

FAILED CARE PACKAGES

Sadly it can be turned off again
And gone in a blink

The minutes, days and years
The laughter and the tears
The hopes and the dreams
The promises over the years

Yet one small detail is missed
The fact it's down to you
To wake up every morning
Correct what others misconstrue

You will champion every minute
Barely have time to think
Ping off emails like clockwork
You don't have time to sink

You alone will plod on
Wonder where you get the strength
But you alone will get there
Because you will go to any length

You will be told you are amazing
Resilient and bold
Or you might be told you are difficult
Whilst your patience is growing old

But you will not give up
No stone will be left unturned
'cause at least you've tried everything
With the research you have learned

You are a carer, mother, father, parent
With a bit between your teeth
And damn those who get in your way
You know who you care for and have belief

You believe in your intuition
You know you can leave your mark
That professionals in ivory towers
Will not leave you in the dark

Be proud for each and every day
That you have struggled through
'cause only you can really know
What life has been like being you!

Six months post the agency being appointed and we were still at the stage of me training staff (this time the agency staff) for staff to leave shortly after being signed off as competent. In the interim one of my remaining night carers handed his notice in after telling Hedge and us that he was hoping to pick up more hours. Hedge was devastated by this announcement as he truly thought, like we did, that this carer would not jump the sinking ship. So within a very few months we had gone down from seven to only two staff and one of those was due to shortly commence her maternity leave. It was wrongly assumed by the care agency that Andrew and I would cover any uncovered shifts on our days off and deliver all the training whilst staff shadowed us. It will therefore come as no surprise to anyone reading this book that I, like others out there, cannot physically work a waking night, get a child to school and work the next day without a break. The carers only ever worked a maximum of two days together or three nights together, yet we were apparently superhuman and could do it all and cope not sleeping in between. The GP asked me during a consultation if I was depressed and if I was eating and sleeping ok. I skirted around the actual issue and told her I was fine. I missed out the minor detail that food consisted of loads of rubbish food like chips, chocolate and other high carb food to keep me awake and that was quick and easy to eat. I also declined to tell her about my sleep pattern being dire. Indeed I was so utterly steamed up when I tried to sleep that I couldn't sleep soundly. This lack of sleep was not helped by the fact that when I was working a waking night shift to care for Hedge, I sometimes had to stay awake the next day to carry on. So if I was being honest with myself I should have said no to both questions. Then again I was not depressed, just exhausted with no hope, therefore my 'no' came easily in my response to the GP.

Christmas was equally vexing due to Hedge needing to be kept in hospital because of the failed care package. Bearing in mind

Hedge was healthy enough to come home and his mental health was deteriorating due to him being so disheartened, Andrew made the decision to take three weeks off work to care for Hedge so he could come home. This decision came from the heart of a selfless man, but the resultant effect had left us with assumed responsibility. But I have to ask you, would you keep your 19 year old son in hospital over Christmas when most years he is in hospital due to being ill, when he was actually in good health this year? I guess in hindsight we would have done the same again, but we were left suffering the consequences to our actions.

The following poem was written for Facebook after dragging ourselves through Christmas and pretending to ourselves that we were doing ok. I was fed up seeing all the happy family photos and stuff saying how wonderful life was, so posted this on some of the support groups I belong to. I truly believe people don't appreciate how much people like me don't need to know how wonderful their lives are. Yes, I know you are all amazing, I just don't need to know every single detail of your amazingly 'normal' family life. Therefore, like me, try to learn to ignore those annoyingly damned irritating festive photographs posted on social media. You are categorically not alone in feeling the irritation of others' enjoyment. I like to ignore their pretend enjoyment, as I very much doubt cleaning up after the 'Elf on a Shelf' or having to constantly think about what the irritating pest is going to get up to next is positively helping anyone enjoy the festive season any more than the next person. So like me try to smile politely when you meet the person whose 'Elf on the Shelf' seems to enjoy itself more than you do at Christmas and think of the time they have wasted creating their festive scenarios for their children to enjoy. I presume I ended up a well-adjusted adult and I never had an 'Elf on the Shelf.' However, one Christmas Eve when I was a child I recall getting into trouble when my sister, brother and me used all the kitchen foil to make fairy wings for a little show we were putting on. None of us could work out why our parents were so cross –– although the little thing of the turkey needing to be cooked might have been a clue. Life was so much simpler for me then, clearly not for my parents who had a turkey in need of cooking and only kitchen foil stuck together using sticky tape and glue to form the shape of fairy wings. I must have been an amazing sugar plum fairy donning silver foil wings. Those were the days...

Christmas and Round Robins

I am glad that Christmas is over
That we survived another year
I am exhausted beyond exhaustion
And will have more to deal with I fear

I have little time for me
I am a robot in disguise

Apart from getting wrinkles
I doubt I am growing wise

I dread my son getting older
I struggle already so bad
It makes my mum heart bleed
And makes me feel so sad

I try to make others listen
I work in a job to give care
But when it comes to me
No-one ever wants to share

So instead I come on here
I can see I am not alone
I can read of other great people
Struggling on their own

So thank you for this group
Thank you for helping me see
Thank you for giving me purpose
To help me be just me!

I won't wish anyone a great new year
I will only wish you peace
That even if just for five minutes
Your worries and struggles will cease

> I only wish that 2019 will bring
> A little bit of hope to you all
> That you can rise above your stresses
> Be proud of achievements and grow tall!

You will be pleased to hear that our self-care came in a delightfully greedy way. There had been a special offer on at our local supermarket for an Irish cream liqueur so we bought four bottles. Over the Christmas period we had pretty much drunk the lot and enjoyed every single drop. No guilt just a few extra holes needed in the belt of my trousers to ensure extra comfort. I am most certainly not advocating drinking alcohol in excess but a little tipple or two is neither here nor there, unless you have a dodgy liver or already like your drink too much (note my little disclaimer in case of any accusations for any bad advice). As for me I shall do what I like as I genuinely don't care and have no-one to blame but myself. Unless of course I can successfully prosecute the Irish cream liqueur company for making their product so delicious that they have coerced me to drink to excess and put on weight. No doubt someone somewhere has already tried to do that and failed, so maybe I shall just stick to buying it on special offer and drinking it when I please. Or has all my letter and email writing finally come in handy –– you choose.

The chance for a new career

I have always held on to the fact that one day Hedge's transition to adult services would happen and I could kick start my nursing career and do something I was extremely passionate about, rather than doing a nursing role because I had no other option. I therefore gave myself six months to find a job that would allow me to achieve something in life that I had long waited for. My new role as Liaison Nurse for Learning Disabilities was a role I had kept an eye on for over two years and when the post came up again I made enquiries and applied for the position. Having seen the job advertised as full time, the advert stated that I could apply for part-time, job share and flexible working. I was shortlisted for interview and nearly pulled out when I saw that the position required me to deliver a presentation to a panel of five professionals. However, I have always had the policy of not letting things pass me by and attended the interview. I was suitably delighted to be offered the position and advised the appointing Manager that I would need to be part-time until my son had completed his transition to adult services. I was fully under the impression that Hedge was about to receive Private Therapy as commissioned by the local community due to them not having the facilities in-house. That was mistake number one. Mistake number two was my belief that working for a department that took pride in caring for people with learning disabilities would actually mean management would have compassion for those that worked there.

It therefore came as a shock to be told by management that work colleagues felt uncomfortable when I talked about my son and that there had been complaints. Fact number one is that I only talked about my son if and when others asked me about him. Fact number two is that I only ever tell people the truth about my life. Fact number three is that I go to work to get away from my caring role, so would have no benefit working and going on about my caring role whilst at work, unless having general chit chat like everyone does in order to make conversation. When I asked who had complained I was basically told that unless an internal investigation was launched then they would not be able to let me know. This did and still does seem rather odd to me, as surely the manager who called me in to tell me of the complaint should have known who it was that they spoke to who had complained. After leaving the office I mulled over the accusation and came to the view that this came from management and was nothing at all to do with my work colleagues. I now regret declining the internal investigation, but at the time felt the whole situation was rather petty. Unsurprisingly, following the accusation about how I had made people feel, I was unable to elicit who could have accused me. Out of the very few people I actually spoke to, they appeared shocked when I told them that management had asked me to not talk about my son at work. It is the first time in my 20 year career as a nurse that I had been accused of this and the whole scenario left me feeling unnerved and on edge and avoiding talking to anyone at all for fear of further accusations. I was also very aware that Andrew had recently put in a concern about the way Hedge's care had been turned down by the service I worked for and it was entirely plausible that this was why I had been told not to talk about Hedge at work.

If I am saying as it is
Don't stab me in the back
As I've feelings too
It's one thing I don't lack

Sadly from where I am
The world ain't a great place
But in order not to offend
I'll paint a smile on my face

I won't bother to say
I won't bother to speak
If the one thing I mention
Makes my world seem bleak

I doubt anyone will notice
If I burn out one day

As it simply won't be their problem
'cause the world just ain't that way!

I am sure this rings a bell with lots of people. I've seen too much of people being sad about how others are behind their backs. Therefore, I just continued to keep smiling and grew thicker rhino skin. Playing devil's advocate though; if something I said did make someone query what they were doing and saying, then surely this should be seen as a good thing as it could elicit change for the better?

Even this situation evoked a self-care moment as I spent longer in the staff toilets contemplating what had been said and spent longer chatting to the nicer people in the department getting to know more about their families and home life. I didn't realise how easy it could be to be a gossip should I have had the inclination to do so. Simply taking a few minutes more to engage in conversation had enabled me to understand some very complex working relationships and I could have caused a riot if I had the energy to do some mud stirring. Fortunately, I am not that type of person, but I can imagine a lot of fun could be caused by asking something that you know might cause combustion to occur. I am certainly not suggesting anyone reading this causes any trouble, but merely that there is pleasure and self-care that can be had from the very thought of it!

Continuing issues at work

My role was to develop services to make reasonable adjustments when providing care to people with learning disabilities. I therefore developed a training package for GP Surgeries and rolled out a newsletter that ran alongside the seasons. I was delighted to be given a positive annual review of my work and efforts. I was verbally told how competently I had managed my work within the reduced working week I was working due to my caring needs and felt that things were on the up. I was therefore not expecting to be called into the manager's office and jointly told by my manager and her manager's manager that my hours that were due to be reviewed could not continue as part-time (albeit 32.5 hours) and had to increase to 37.5 hours. Apparently they needed more of me not less and had been 'cut to the bone due to lack of funding and couldn't afford to lose anymore clinical hours'. I sat there in shock and after the very brief meeting politely left the office, went to my office, broke down in tears and left. Fortunately, I had annual leave the following day and my nursing union representative and Occupational Health encouraged me to seek alternative work. Their fears were that if I did try to work full-time hours I might have ended up in breach of my contract or wreck my career as the result of a disciplinary due to not being in a position to fulfil the contracted hours.

I very much doubt that management appreciated why I was compelled to seek alternative employment. Sadly it was due to being unable to work the full-time hours as a direct result of a failed transition to adult services that happened to be the same organisation that I worked for. In fact it was the same Locality Manager who told me about my hours and told me that I had to separate out my caring role from my working role, who was chairing meetings regarding Hedge's failed transition to adult services. I felt let down, sad, empty and like a boat sailing into the unknown without a rudder.

>Empty and hollow
>How do you describe?
>When feeling like this
>Feels deeper inside
>
>Empty no hope
>How do you think?
>When tears are near
>And you feel on the brink
>
>Empty and alone
>How do you say?
>When you only smile
>And say you're ok

'THE UNOFFICIAL SELF-CARE GUIDE FOR CARERS'

You are not depressed
You don't need a hug
You just need a break
A hot drink in a mug

You are exhausted
Tired of the constant fight
Just needing action
And support as a right

Your body is weary
Not from depression inside
But from constant alertness
And roller coaster ride

You want to get off
You can't as you care
You just want a system
That is truthful and fair

You don't want the pity
The pat on the back
You just want honesty
To help keep you on track

Your sigh is from within
Hope fading fast

Wondering how long
Your exhaustion will last

You see others going out
Yet can't quite join in
'cause you never stop caring
And see self-care as a sin

Yet like me you do need self-care
Time to recover, to keep banging the drum
To start the day over yet again
And carry on just being mum!

So I was forced to re-evaluate my life at a time when I was also being increasingly expected to cover the gaps in care. My hope of finding alternative employment seemed doomed as nothing seemed to be quite what I was looking for. However, I knew that in order to manage my own self-care I needed to find something, otherwise I would be dragged deeper into providing constant backup care for Hedge.

I was well and truly trapped in a situation that could leave me jobless and having to care for free as I didn't qualify for anything to help me financially in my caring role. My rights appeared not to exist and the government was about to wave goodbye to another nurse who couldn't work due to the crazy situation that I had been put in. Not to mention the fact that the team where I had been working was quite prepared to go without anyone in post (for many months) whilst they attempted to recruit, rather than enable me to work 4.5 hours less each week. Even now I cannot understand their logic, as roll on a year and I could have increased my working hours to full-time.

(As a point of note: after leaving the Learning Disability Team I bumped into numerous members of the team and some of the newest ex-employees, who have openly told me that they were sad that I had left and were appalled at the way I had been treated -- which adds to my belief that the accusations about me came from management, possibly due to me having insider knowledge of the way the team accepted people to their service.)

Every cloud has a silver lining and my silver lining was being forced to re-evaluate my working life due to the way I had been treated. If I had not worked for the Learning Disability Team I could not have applied for my current role. I do believe in fate and wonder if this was fate playing its part again like it did when I ended up working at a Private Hospital after being severely bullied in my previous role as a Cashier at a Building Society. The Matron of the Private Hospital had queried my short length of service with another employee of the hospital who had previously worked at the same Building Society and the staff member (whom I had never met) put in a good word for me.

Therefore, like me you might get a silver lining in your cloud. If you don't then put up your brolly or wear a hat, as when the rain clouds open you will need to be protected from the deluge. I therefore have a brolly stand in my hallway and keep a hat handy to slap on my head for when I am having a particularly bad hair day; this easily doubles up as something for my daughter to vomit in if she is ever car sick. Thus preventing you from having to spend ages trying to scrub your car clean and get rid of the odour of vomit from your car. Gosh aren't you glad you are reading this book with all the helpful hints within it! Whilst I am on a roll regarding handy tips, Bicarbonate of Soda does wonders for soaking up urine from car footwells. I used about six tubs of it following the unfortunate incident of a catheter bag tap opening in my car's footwell. It was a dark wet Friday evening so I quickly mopped up the mess when I arrived home. I then forgot all about it until I went to use the car the following Monday. It is safe to say that I was not expecting the odour that travelled up my nostrils when I got in the car and I nearly needed my hat to vomit in myself. Fortunately, a Social Worker who happened to be visiting that day mentioned about using Bicarbonate of Soda, so I bought a load and threw it in the car. This mercifully did the trick in drying up the carpet but I didn't quite fancy using my vacuum cleaner to clean up the resultant dried mess. I therefore have a small confession to make as I used one from the local garage. I did clean the end of the nozzle after using it and my car ended up no longer smelling like the inside of a public toilet. I even managed a bit of self-care time too, as it wasn't me who vacuumed the car but Andrew as he told me I wasn't putting enough effort into doing it. It works every time as I have mastered very nicely how not to put enough effort into a lot of things in order for Andrew to show me how things are done properly. Yes, self-care can unquestionably be most rewarding. This tactic can also be utilized in other situations –– the possibilities are endless so long as you can keep a deadpan face if your motives are ever delved into any further.

Here we go again

In the first six months of the first care agency starting, we had: one carer that never turned up; another that turned up and left shortly after he was signed off as he decided claiming benefits was easier; another who would be great but also worked on another package of care and was not interested in doing any extra hours; another who was meant to be working nights but decided that she did not want to do nights anymore and gave Hedge a leave date of two weeks; another who was lovely but couldn't work nights as she falls asleep at 04:00 hours (I have to add that so would I if I did not take my Pro Plus and also drink copious amounts of caffeine all night long, that then renders me too wide awake to sleep in the morning); another who was and still is a Professional Golfer (again lovely, but in reality was going to be off playing golf once he got a sponsorship); oh and another one who turned up late to her first two live shifts and deemed it was funny to tell Hedge she was a murderer (so Hedge understandably said he did not want her back as he did not trust her). Deep joy not. Individually they were all great (apart from the murderer who had apparently been in prison and the other carer who was now claiming benefits in preference to working who had also told Hedge he had been in prison), but between them they could not cover the shifts, so the agency were back to recruiting yet again and I was expected to once again cover more shifts as a freebie.

So was I anxious? Yes I was anxious and exhausted and getting fatter, greyer and more wrinkly and stiff in the joints whilst I waited patiently for time for me.

Anxiety and its consequences

Anxious for stillness
Anxious for life
Anxious for anything
That doesn't give me strife

Anxious a knot so deep
Anxious a weight to wear
Anxious to please
And wanting to care

Anxious to sleep
Anxious to wake
Anxious to find solace
And to give more than to take

Anxious to see the reason
Anxious to see through the trees
Anxious to find laughter
And not in despair on my knees

Anxious to make it right
Anxious to just get through the day
Anxious to be just me
And allowed to be only that way

And to add to my anxiety Hedge was still not getting the mental health support or therapy he so desperately needed and questions were still being asked about his IQ.

Will I? Can I? Shall I try?
Take each day and not ask why
Do I? Could I? May I?
See flying pigs in the sky!

Take the risk or lose the chance
Be walked over or take a stance
Sit and wonder what if and why?
Others have rainbows in the sky!

Should I stand up, be proud and tall?
Or should I sit down and take a fall?
Am I a mouse, not rearing up high?
Shelter from rain or create thunder in the sky!

I am me, take me or leave me
I can't be like others so just let me be
I struggle to ride the storm, I cannot lie
My relaxing days are just pie in the sky

I work hard, I rarely go off sick
I can sort out problems and think real quick
If others don't like it I don't need to know why
'cause they are the clouds in my sky

Don't pretend you know me
Don't think I can't really see
'cause fake friends I don't easily buy
My real friends are the sun in my sky

My friends don't gossip, they don't leave me out
My friends understand me even when I say nowt
My friends just get it and don't judge or even try
They are the angels in my cloud darkened sky!

Yet again enforced self-care meant eating chips, pot noodles and anything easy like a pasty or pie to get the carbs I so desperately constantly craved. If Hedge ever fell asleep during the day I would grab the remote control and flick through the channels for ten minutes before having yet more self-care by way of tidying around. This also counted as my exercise as I tend to get a tiny bit puffed out vacuuming and reaching for the cobwebs is counted as my stretches. There are just so many inventive ways to get a good workout and exercise that I have also convinced myself I have no need to go to the gym. Therefore saving money on the membership and having more money in my pocket to buy those greasy simply decadent nibbles called chips.

The curious case of being Hedge

Hedge was born with a rare chromosome abnormality and has suffered many medical errors and misdiagnoses that have led to him being like he is. It is unclear what impacts on what or what affects what. But what is clear is that Hedge is unique and will never fit the boxes that society and the medical profession want him to fit into. The one thing that is plainly clear is that there is no service out there that can meet his needs, which is why at the age of almost 21, we are still attempting to get Hedge the care he needs. There are also some very sloping shouldered people out there prepared to spin and spin again in order to not provide a service to Hedge (even though commissioned reports by the local health authority firmly directed towards a service being provided).

The relentless management of Hedge's escalated anxieties alongside attendance at meetings and meeting numerous different professionals continued to achieve nothing. It was very much taking one step forward and four steps back.

Within a period of just a few days Hedge sustained a burn to the back of his neck from a hot wheat bag, had to attend a clinic and have a load of Entonox for pain relief due to his catheter being pulled, had another incident report completed due to him having a chest of drawers fall on him (Hedge was trying to fix a knob he had accidentally pulled off). Quite why Hedge decided to sit in the drawer in order to fix the knob remains a mystery to us all. And so it goes on. Not a day passed by without yet another oddity that no-one could quite explain, yet these obscurities added to the list of concerns.

This combined with the growing list of other things Hedge had instigated, such as putting his house on the market for £2000.00 believing it was a lot of money. I had a bidding war of people phoning me up offering to pay cash. As Hedge rented the property, the house was not his to sell. It downheartedly made me wonder what kind of people were assuming anyone was putting a house on the market for only £2000.00 or were they just preying on Hedge's miscalculation?

At long last Hedge purchased his 3D TV which he said was his life-long dream; this was TV number four and was second hand from a local charity shop. Hedge next wanted a cat. Hedge seemed to forget that our large ginger tomcat (Borry) went between both houses and was already his cat. In the summer I reluctantly caved in and helped him purchase a guinea pig that sadly had to be rehomed after Hedge was in hospital for 14 weeks and lost interest in it. On the plus side it did stop

Hedge going on about wanting to be a vet or zookeeper as he realised the guinea pig needed daily care and was rather time consuming. I dreaded to think what it would be next. I rather hoped that I could avoid the cat as due to the amount of time Hedge spent ill, I could only guess who would be left looking after it.

I had limited time for self-care as it was, let alone caring for another pet. Although according to research it is scientifically proven (apparently) that having a pet and stroking it can help relax you and help you to live for longer. That is what I have heard anyway! Fish are also meant to be relaxing, although my mother's fish got a lump on it and needed a lot of money spending on it and a great deal of time messing about with cleaning the tank etc. Therefore, a pet like a cat that pretty much cared for itself seemed not too bad to me. Andrew would rather have had a dog, but I liked to think of all the time I was saving by not having to walk it. If I added up all these hours that might have been wasted walking a dog, then goodness what a lot of spare time I might have. Only I didn't have the extra time I might have saved because I worked and was a carer and mum and wife and so the list went on. So, a cat was sounding like a better option each time I endeavoured to think of an alternative. Famous last words…

Time

Time to sit and reflect
Time to ponder on
Time to wonder why
And where the time has gone

Time to rush around
Time to sit and think
Time not to watch the telly
As the TV's on the blink

Time to enjoy the sunshine
Time to get outdoors
Time to sweep up leaves
Before the other chores

Time for me and self-care
Time to chill out and be me
Time to hide in the bathroom
No-one can hear or see

Time for just a little break
Time to take a breath
Time to be mum again
Before I'm worked to death

Time for just five minutes
Time just a moment in space
Time to care for the children
Who flourish at their own time and pace

Time to really appreciate
Time to know what is mine
Time to stop for just a minute
Knowing I am doing just fine

Time to not feel eternally guilty
Time to see that to prevent a fall
Time is needed to appreciate just me
'cause without 'me time' I can't do it all!

Thinking of others before myself

I have struggled daily to understand the concept of self-care and whole heartedly believe it is the part of me that is a nurse through and through, and for me it is a vocation. Combine my role as a mother and my commitment to parenthood that goes beyond that given by an average parent and there is little wonder that I have time to worry, but worry I do. I have a child who has struggled to be accepted, ignored by many and either loved or hated like Marmite. Andrew thinks that it is stress that causes me to worry unnecessarily about others and their own plights, rather than walking by. I see it as a need to stand up for them and do all I can to help in the limited time I have available. During the winter months I spend time worrying about those without roofs over their heads and homeless having to sleep in shop doorways. How many of us just walk on by trying to not make eye contact. I do buy the Big Issue and watched the film 'A Street Cat Named Bob'. For me it is yet another example where society has failed. Yes, people make their own way in life, but no-one knows anyone's story or the reason for the person being homeless. I recall a nurse who worked at the same organization as me explaining about the 'Wake and Shake' project she was part of. I never knew that she worked outside of her day job and went away after our talk thinking very differently about this unassuming nurse.

> When the nights are drawing in
> And there is more darkness than daylight
> Think of the poor souls sleeping in a doorway
> Cold and no roof over head or warmth in sight
>
> When you dash to your car
> Freezing from the rain
> Think of the poor souls
> Wishing they had a home again
>
> When you snuggle up
> Warm drink close by
> Think of the poor souls
> Wondering how and why
>
> Why have they ended up here?
> Why are they alone?
> Why do they have no warmth?
> And no place to call home?
>
> Why do people just walk by?
> And pretend not to see
> Ignore the cold blue hands
> Just letting them be

So if you do one good thing
Think of those out there
Those who fell into homelessness
Who want to love and share

Look for solutions not excuses,
Don't ignore and bury your head
Find a way to support where you can
So a vulnerable person can find a bed

I suppose I have a heart, but my heart is growing tired and frustrated as a result of all the excuses made by those who are meant to care. I am sure I am not alone. Conversely if I do someone a good deed it does make me feel inherently better in myself and give me a lift. Giving can be so much more rewarding than receiving. Although personally I do not find being a carer is rewarding in any way shape or form. Being a carer is certainly more about giving than receiving. I just want to be mum, being mum is hard enough. Therefore on my Birthday and at Christmas I give myself one present I know I want but what I know no-one will give me even though I have hinted for months. This way I get the reward of receiving and giving. If only all other self-care could be so easy to resolve. I then smile smugly to myself about the memory of when Andrew purchased me the necklace with a pendant that disappeared down my non-existent cleavage and looked like something you might find in a bric-a-brac stall, the wallpaper stripper or the numerous other ill-conceived ideas of a thought-provoking presents. I innocently say, "Oh isn't that lovely I wonder who bought it for me?"

Self-care Support Groups

Having surfed Facebook I have joined several groups under my assumed name. My own page gives only information that is not confidential, a few photos, mainly links and poems that have been written to help others in their caring roles. Some are not about me and my life, but poems I have been asked to write by others who I know and I have therefore chosen to share these to a wider audience.

Two such groups I belong to are Self-care support groups that encourage people like me to not feel guilty for taking time to self-care. As explained in my previous book you can't pour from an empty cup and as I often feel like a sponge that can't take anymore and will start dripping its load if one more thing is added to my daily struggles, I need to respect my time out. Even when bearing that in mind, I also find it incredibly hard to justify time out for me to have five minutes to relax. When at home I feel bad if I am not cleaning, decluttering or sorting the garden. In a way this is my self-care; however, I end up exhausted and contented as I have been able to focus on something other than Hedge.

Give me a moment please

Just one day is all I want
An hour would be great
Five minutes to not stress and worry
But that's clearly not my fate

Instead each and every day
A new disaster does appear
East Enders couldn't write a better script
Roll on the next damn year

I don't want my lot in life
I didn't choose disability
I got it dumped upon my lap
And now it's my reality

No-one can really understand
Ever appreciate or even know
What lies behind my mask
Who really cares if I am low?

I do my best for my patients
I give great advice for learning too
As for me it never really works
I simply don't have a clue

'THE UNOFFICIAL SELF-CARE GUIDE FOR CARERS'

I've tried it all, I've listened hard
I email, chase and telephone
But without the correct support
I might as well be on my own

Those in power don't seem to care
They've budgets to manage I know
So who really cares if my child
Deteriorates to a new state of low

Let's battle who funds it
Let's write another report
Let's fob off the parents with an email
Let's see the time we've bought

We'll procrastinate and rearrange
We'll copy in the boss
'cause once 5pm arrives
We couldn't give a toss

We're off home it's the weekend
We'll leave the parents going insane
Who cares if they're worried sick
We'll pass the buck again

When Monday comes the email box
Well it's full of 'oh so much'

> We'll ping off an email
> Saying 'We'll soon be in touch'
>
> And before you know it
> Another week has flown by
> And wonders never cease
> Flying pigs are even in the sky
>
> I am done with worrying
> I am done with caring
> I am done with wishing
> My hair beyond the tearing!
>
> Will someone please respond
> Make a decision and see
> It's not just my son that needs help
> It's also MEEEEEEE!

So there we have it, do I really count? Does anyone out there really care about the carer? A person or professional can make all the correct 'arhh', 'you are amazing', 'you are so good' etc noises, but as far as I can tell it is mainly piecemeal and amounts to not a lot in action. Andrew and I thought we were having a Carer's Assessment completed but nothing materialised; I gave up waiting as the Social Worker who was allocated to do this seemed to have vanished from the face of the planet. I somehow managed to arrange another person to complete the assessment and then annoyingly the initial Social Worker came back to say that she could visit a few days before the one I had managed to arrange. I ended up turning down the assessment from the initial Social Worker as she worked where I did and at the time I feared that there would be a conflict of interest should I dare speak to her and I did not wish to open a can of worms or put her in a compromised situation. So just like buses, you wait and wait and wait and then two arrive at once. Although sadly I doubted that having a Carer's Assessment completed would do anything to alleviate the situation we found ourselves in. History cannot be undone, and it is the history for Hedge that we are trying to rewrite and make better through therapy that is simply not there to be had. *(By way of an update, five months later neither Andrew or myself had received a copy of either of our Carer's Assessments that we were promised upon completion of our appointments with the respective Social Workers.)*

It's got to be the most miserable job just completing Carer's Assessments all day, as I am pretty certain that not many carers say what a fun time they are having. On the plus side, having the Carer's Assessment did mean that I was forced to sit down and whinge on for an hour or two about why life is so challenging. I even got to have two cups of coffee and opened a new pack of biscuits. I'll politely forget about all the chasing I had to do in order to get the Carer's Assessment arranged. I dread to think how many years of my life has been sent chasing. In spite of this I would still strongly promote the value of a Carer's Assessment as it is a document that highlights the extra work you do and may help towards additional support or enable you to apply for a Carer's Card as evidence for free or reduced price entry when accompanying the person you are caring for on a rare trip out. That's if you have enough energy to want to go for a rare trip out. Most importantly it is very satisfying to see all you do written down, especially knowing that someone else has had to sit there and listen to you tell your story (it was for me anyway) and I will happily wave it at anyone who dares question my role as a carer.

Friends and the great escape

I have retained only a few friends since having Hedge and the local carers groups that are meant to support seem to forget that some carers work whilst juggling care needs and also have other children that serve to isolate carers further whilst undertaking the caring role.

I have two long distance friends who keep me sane and we spend many hours on the phone supporting each other.

I also meet a very small group of ladies who I met when we had Little sis.

I am eternally grateful for having these people in my life as without them I doubt I would have kept the sense of humour and sense of reality that I have. Together we guide each other through the challenges of life and one of my friends has struggled more than most and I admire her each and every day when I think of the challenges she has faced since her husband left her. I know I could not have managed my situation if I did not have Andrew by my side, and I dread it when he goes abroad for work, as I can guarantee there will be some disaster and I will be left spinning plates all in one go.

If I dare hope to escape for a rare evening out, then someone or something transpires that prevents it from happening. I do get pangs of jealousy when I think of Andrew breaking free from the monotony, as I have not had a break away to do with work or otherwise for nearly five years now. That's if I don't count when I took Little sis away for a few nights last summer. So the fact Andrew has been off to Dubai or Saudi for work makes me a tad green with envy, actually rather a bright emerald green with envy. The likelihood of me utilising my passport and escaping remained and continues to remain non-existent. Whilst I appreciated Andrew was working, the working away did enable him to have the evenings free, not forgetting the weekends free, which rarely happened for me. Each time Andrew went away it seemed to coincide with some disaster that I was forced to resolve. More often than not it involved me working back-to-back shifts due to the care agency unexpectedly losing members of staff. Therefore, the idea of no sleep and also caring for a bored younger child never filled my heart or mind with many happy thoughts. Deep joy not, especially when the last few years had taken its toll and if I could I would have happily walked, but couldn't as I have a conscience. Although it does make me appreciate just why so many marriages and relationships break up when couples are having to constantly manage the stress and anxiety of a child who has complications whilst also having to juggle other childcare, work and home life issues. I am pretty sure that I am not alone in my views.

At least when at work my own nightmare could be ignored, as I was focusing on something else instead. Sorting out everyone else's problems was so much easier than sorting out my own life. Yep life has a habit of currently going one way only and more than once I have officially hit the bottom. As a colleague said to me in jest "There is only one way you can go when you hit the bottom –– along." It took me a moment to appreciate what she meant. When the truth of what she said dawned I clearly visualised myself just wading through the mud at the bottom whilst I desperately attempted to seek any peaks towards the positives. Like so many other carers, I desperately need the chance for an escape and struggle when there is nothing but nothingness on the horizon.

I look back and realise that not only have I had a married life of 27 years but for a good 21 of that I have had nothing but worry and stress whilst championing the cause of Hedge, carers and other children/young adults. Self-care now comes alongside humour, I am happy to smile and laugh, quite often at myself and my own life situation. It creates laughter lines (not wrinkles) and a wise head that means I don't give a monkey's about what others might think when I am in mother bear mode. Self-praise is no praise and I certainly don't praise myself for anything other than for trying and being brave enough to smile at myself!

I looked in the mirror
And what do I see

Fine lines and wrinkles
Looking back at me

My eyes once bright
With a glint and shine
Now looking dull and hollow
Those brown eyes of mine

I was never vain
So no need to despair
But look at me now
With stubborn grey hair

My eyeliner seems
Far darker than I need
My age spots are even
Appearing at speed

What happened to me?
Where exactly did I go?
I apply the wonder cream
Hoping the shadows won't show

Most people like summer
I dread its return
As I've only flabby flesh
That prefers to just burn

My feet don't look bad
In fact I am quite proud
But why oh why thread veins
Surely they aren't allowed?

OK there are my boobs
With those I'm quite glad
That they only sag slightly
And don't look too sad

So I pile on the anti-aging cream
Eyeliner, lipstick in place
And escape for the night
With my tired looking face

I guess I only have myself to blame
'cause I can't be bothered to colour again
The roots looked worse when peeking through
And the harshness of colour just liked to stain

For now I am proud, I am grey
It's the new colour that's in
Only my colour is natural
It really is all win-win!

Oh dear I am not sure if I do like the grey, but worrying about the pesky coarse grey hairs peeking through my hairline was more stressful than bothering and wasting time trying to colour my hair every few weeks. The thing that worries me the most is the wrinkles. My mother always told me that failing eyesight was a positive as it meant you wouldn't mind so much about your wrinkles. I always said I wouldn't bother with Botox but it does sound more appealing the more wrinkled and dry my face continues to become. The only problem is the slight issue of the cost and the fact I don't like injections. So I will cheerfully count my blessings for the fact that I now need to wear glasses to be able to see my face clearly in the mirror and as I often can't find where I have left my glasses I am fairly safe at not feeling depressed each time I pass a reflective surface.

I once used to watch a programme on the TV that aged people if they continued with their current lifestyle. I am curious as to what Andrew and I would look like now if we had not had the constant challenges of parenting and caring for Hedge and his complex needs. Maybe I should write to the BBC to ask them to do that series. You never know, it might get excellent ratings and even make those who have the power to make a change eventually see the damage that having limited support and constant challenges with no chance of escape does to your body! I can see it now, not 'Escape to the Country', but 'Escape your Caring Role'. I can live and dream. My self-care hint –– buy a bucketful of hair bands, grow your hair and tie it back. You will take years of your worn out, sleep deprived face and instantly look younger without the need for an expensive face lift or face cream. If you tie your hair back too tight you might suffer the risk or having a slightly surprised look as your eyebrows are pulled high up, but at least you will be wearing the look fittingly should some help possibly come your way. Alternatively buy some more nails and rehang your mirrors higher up so that when you look in them you have to stretch your neck up to view your face. Trust me, this does work as being vertically challenged I've already had the good fortune to utilise this trick many times before. Just be careful though not to hammer a nail into an electrical cable otherwise you might also be donning a new curly hairdo!

Guinea pig trials

I know I want an easy life, and sometimes have had to give in for a moment of peace and quiet, but sadly my decision to not say a firm no landed me knee deep in straw. Hedge's continual need to purchase high ticketed goods took a different direction and he decided he needed a pet to keep him company. I was reluctant for another cat due to ours already going between houses and I did not want to put his nose out of joint. So what better way to appease Hedge than to agree to him having a small animal in a cage? I have only had a rabbit as a child and know that this was a burden for my own mother due to me and my siblings growing tired of looking after the rabbits after a few weeks. Sounds familiar to anyone –– I am sure it does. So on yet another day of caring for Hedge I was conned into taking him to a Pet Shop and we checked out the smaller rodents like hamsters. It was soon pretty obvious that a hamster would not be appropriate due to Hedge's poor hand-eye co-ordination and that he could kill it by inadvertently dropping it. Deep joy not as we moved on to the bigger rodents like rats and guinea pigs. I know some people find rats endearing but there is something I really don't like about their skinny bald tails, sharp teeth and claws. I therefore agreed to look at the guinea pigs. Hedge was so excited that he was having difficulty staying still in his wheelchair and he was even more delighted when the guinea pig was popped lovingly on his lap. Now bearing in mind this is the first time I have touched a guinea pig since having one as a class pet in the 1970s, I was a tad concerned about caring for it. Yes I appreciate the guinea pig was meant to be for Hedge, but being honest with myself I knew it was going to be down to my dear self to care for it when the carers failed to turn up or when Hedge was in hospital, which is where he spends an awful lot of time residing.

Oh my goodness I hadn't even realised that guinea pigs had such huge cages either. As the guinea pig was on his own due to the previous one he was sharing with attacking him, we were advised that we should buy a larger cage. "Great," said through pursed lips, a 1.5 metre long cage, a bale of hay for bedding, a huge quantity of specialised feed, vitamin drops, bowl, house, water bottle later and so the list went on, £185.00 lighter we left carrying the guinea pig in a stripy cardboard box. Quite how I squeezed everything into the car is remarkable when the wheelchair takes up most of the boot. So I get Hedge home, wheelchair out, guinea pig out, cage etc out and put it all together in Hedge's house. I only had to break the news to the carers and kept my fingers and toes crossed that none of them would complain too loudly about their additional chores. One of the newest carers was scared of guinea pigs and looked like she was putting her hand in a box of hand eating spiders each time she cleaned the cage out, another got urine all over himself the first time he took the guinea pig out for a cuddle and another felt that we did not have enough to stimulate him. Therefore in only a very few weeks the guinea pig named Rolo had toys, tunnels, nibbles to hang from the side of the cage and puppy training pads to pop on the lap of anyone who wanted a cuddle to prevent urine going everywhere.

The house smelt like a barn and the bin was full to overflowing of wood shavings from the toileting habits of the guinea pig, as the guinea pig decided he did not wish to use the corner toilet tray I was also advised to purchase.

In the first month the guinea pig racked up a huge food bill too, as he only liked spinach, blueberries, strawberries and kale and was not too keen on his dried guinea pig food. How the heck can something so small be so damn fussy? Trust Hedge to have a picky eater. I soon became very aware that the guinea pig was eating more healthily than me and I had absolutely no idea how noisy they were. Rolo was cute at first, but then every time I moved it would start squeaking for food and making me feel guilty by poking its tiny delicate paws through the cage bars trying desperately to get my attention. Couple this with the fact that Hedge was having an epic long stay in hospital meant that Rolo had to move into my Kitchen/Diner. According to Andrew the guinea pig loved it when I walked into the room and he kindly told me that it showed that I was also bonding with him. Hmmm, not quite how I saw it. According to what I googled Guinea pigs always squeaked when they hear their owners as it is a way to get them to feed them and whilst it may have appeared I was bonding that was simply not true. Believe me, spending time bending in through the top of a humungous 1.5 metre cage and scooping out wood shaving full of excrement was not exactly my idea of self-care. Neither was doing a dash to sit down sporting a puppy training pad on my lap, hoping that the little fellow was not going to pass urine all over the mat and the mat to leak on me or far worse that the guinea pig was now sitting in its own excrement and I had to do a dash to get the guinea pig back to his cage. As far as self-care was concerned, I was having the chance to sit down and cuddle a vaguely cute furry animal, whilst Borry glared at me from the other side of my patio doors pawing at the windows to be let in. I also had to remind myself to clean mud off the windows where Borry had tried frantically to alert my attention to get in, whilst I was busy trying to pretend he was not there whilst providing the guinea pig a bit of cuddle time.

In the meantime, Hedge had all but forgotten he ever had a guinea pig and had not mentioned him once. All I knew is that I was now paying for the food, hay, wood shavings etc and spending time twice a day cleaning Rolo out. I daren't ask Hedge if he wanted to re-home him and was locked in the situation like so many other parents are when their children decide their pet they were so desperate for is no longer interesting. I had clearly been a complete mug to agree to the guinea pig in the first place and had only myself to blame.

Roll on 14 weeks in hospital and Hedge only mentioned the guinea pig twice and that was after I took photos of it to show Hedge. Therefore I decided to rehome him. Interestingly Hedge was grateful at this idea as he called poor Rolo a smelly little rodent. I could have crowned Hedge and Hedge knew I was far from impressed, especially when Hedge told me that I should have rehomed him earlier. I fortunately managed to rehome him quite quickly and even drove the cage and all the bits to the person's house and Andrew and I made a quick escape once Rolo was in their arms. I did feel a tad guilty, but looking at the whole experience positively, my house no longer smelt of hay and Rolo did serve a purpose in that Hedge was no longer going on about being a Zookeeper.

The trouble was that this only proved to foster Hedge's pleas for a cat as he told me that Borry did not spend enough time in his house. Once again I felt myself being sucked right in and this time Hedge knew that if he lost interest in a cat then I would be mug enough to take another cat on as I simply adore cats.

> To all those out there
> Who are conned into getting a pet
> Don't give in just stand your ground
> Or for years you will regret
>
> Be it furry rodent or the reptile kind
> You will be sure to be the one

Who cares for it and cleans it out
Whilst your kids sit on their bum

We are told that pets are great
They teach about loving and care
But in my view some caged pets
Just teach me how to swear

Each time I saw the cage
Poor Rolo gave a squeak
I'd get him out for a cuddle
And see his bladder leak

Hay all around the kitchen
Wood shavings on the floor
Nibbles and bits of parsley
And wooden things to gnaw

I could have kept a horse
For what poor Rolo cost
So I was grateful to rehome
Not sad for the money that I've lost

I hope his new home is happier
Now he lives elsewhere
'cause five minute wonders
On caged animals just ain't fair!

My dilemma was that Borry was very territorial and might not bond with a new cat. Predictably I could feel myself being well and truly conned into getting one. I could just imagine how calming a cat could be around the house and great company for Hedge too. All for a quiet life or was it??

Even this situation had self-care entwined within it. My house had been looking cluttered when I had all the guinea pig's bits and pieces taking up every spare corner and once it was all gone I could be proud of my 'space' where the clutter used to be. I could also sit in peace and quiet and munch on the leftover spinach and carrot sticks that I forgot to give the new owner.

A child's answers to our prayers

"Think Hedge is much younger and then you won't feel so cross," says nine year old Little sis. Thanks, Little sis, that made me feel down in the dumps that you had worked out a way for getting on so agreeably with your big brother and I was coping and managing so badly. Well they do say out of the mouths of babes and she did and continues to speak a lot of sense.

My newest self-care talk to myself involved me telling myself to not get so het up about things that I used to do at 19 years old and feeling guilty about what Hedge can and can't do at a similar age. Whilst I had a job at the age of 15, passed my driving test at 17 and went out to pubs and nightclubs, even working in both during my late teens to supplement my full time job's income, this has not been possible for Hedge. Realistically this was not ever going to happen for Hedge unless he was accompanied by a carer/support worker, so I needed to chill out and recognise Hedge was just Hedge, no more, no less. I think what didn't help was the constant battle to get people to recognise that Hedge actually had a problem as when they met Hedge briefly he could talk the talk which resulted in first impressions never being correct. So there we had it, a self-care talk regarding my need as a parent to not feel bad about where Hedge was in his life and that included ignoring those who were bigoted towards Hedge. I hoped to learn to accept Hedge as he was and enjoy being mum and not constantly beating myself up over what could have been and should be happening right now. It was not going to help me have peace with myself and it was due to the way the services had failed him so badly. Therefore, get real, get a life and eat more chips to pacify myself. See that was easy, wasn't it? Buy a bag of chips with plenty of vinegar and light on the salt and I can take on the world. My cholesterol level can go on hold for now.

In the meantime, Little sis may continue to help me enjoy 'Slothikins' (as kindly named by Little sis) by using her ways of thinking and coping.

> My brother has a wheelchair
> My brother has a smirky grin
> My brother has smiley eyes
> He has sticky out hair and chin
>
> My brother can be annoying
> My brother can be loud
> My brother gives me cuddles
> He also makes me proud

My brother's just unique
My brother's just like me
My brother's protective
He shouts if I climb a tree

My brother calls me 'Green furry' (as in monster)
My brother calls me loud
My brother loves me to pieces
He says I make him proud

My brother can be poorly
My brother can get sick
My brother goes to hospital
To make him better quick

My brother is amazing
My brother makes people smile
My brother has carers
So mum can rest a while

Maybe this is just what the Occupational Therapist was alluding to all those years ago when she told me to have another child. It has only taken me 15 years to work out what she meant. So, let's all have more children so they can then do the caring, what a simply fantastic idea. If only I had known 15 years ago, I could have had a houseful of children to make my life easier.

Planning for the future

Admittedly it is not the sort of thing most people decide to do, but we did a lot of thinking regarding what might happen after we are no longer here. We eventually made our wills after many years procrastinating. This decision was prompted after realising we no longer needed to press gang people into being Hedge's guardian due to him no longer being a child. We therefore appointed a firm of Solicitors who were also appointed as the Executors of the will (for a fee). However, after I am dead I really don't care if the Solicitors will be charging a fee for this, as at least it is sorted.

Andrew and I have also decided on a Funeral Plan. We just need to decide on who will do it. I have even written my own Epitaph as I have no wish for people to pretend I was something I have not been after I am dead. I want people to know the real me. I would far rather dispense of the need for a funeral so that I can do away with people pretending they are upset when the coffin arrives. Who likes funerals in any case and in my view too many people interfere and the wake afterwards only serves to bring people together who have not met for years. On the plus side, due to the fact that I don't have a social life or masses of friends and now don't even have work colleagues to count on attending, it should be a quiet affair. So being a carer does have its plus side and whilst I reside in my coffin I will finally be having the well-earned rest I have desired for such a long time. OK so maybe I am being just a tiny bit morbid, but be honest, has this thought not also crossed your mind? I have been to funerals with mourners packed to the rafters. Have they truly all been great friends of the deceased or just filled full of morbid curiosity? Maybe I will never know, but mine will be small. I could probably count on 15 - 20 people attending, and that is if some of those have not snuffed it before me.

As for my box, I would like a nice non-complex neat box, maybe made of willow and I would like to dispense with the cars so that people can arrive when I am already at the crematorium. I detest being late and going slow along a road would drive me batty, whilst my poor relatives sit crying in the back of another car. I appreciate I am assuming they will be crying, they will probably be thinking to themselves 'Thank God she's gone, the moany old bat.' I certainly don't need to be carried in on the shoulders of a random mix of different height relatives either, all near to collapsing due to my weight. I will get the minister (if I must have one) say the words I have written. I would not put my children in the dire situation of gulping back tears whilst saying anything. Then I would like a nice rousing song to see me out. Prefab Sprout – King of Rock and Roll should do the trick as it reminds me of lovely hot summers in the 1980s when I was still young enough to not worry too much. I love that song, not many other people have the same emotions about the song, but I am confident that it might raise a smile or two as people sit wondering if the minister has put on the correct song. Actually whilst proofreading this book I now also rather like Tones and I - Dance Monkey (but I am not sure about the lyrics as I certainly would not want to do all this caring malarkey all again). In any case "Ta Dah", funeral sorted. Then afterwards for my best meal ever 'Fish and Chips', at a local pub (that's if any pubs still exist by then). I have also recently seen adverts on the television about Pure Cremations, what a great idea, maybe I shall just scrap all the above and look into that instead!

My main wish is to be cremated; I have no desire to be dug up by some Archaeologist in years to come. The thought of a future Archaeologist getting anyone to recreate my body in clay and sticking me in a museum thousands of years from now, fills me with dread.

> Choosy I might be
> But I like to get it right
> Funerals are costly
> And I'm a little tight
>
> So if I plan it carefully
> It need not cost a lot
> 'cause when I'm not here
> I will soon be long forgot

'THE UNOFFICIAL SELF-CARE GUIDE FOR CARERS'

There will be no headstone
Pretending I was great
No flowers saying mum
Or mourners in a state

I want it quick and simple
To be there before the mob
One quick song to say goodbye
Whilst my children sob

A quickie wake to eat
Fish and chips then strawberries and cream
That way those mourners won't think
That Andrew's being mean

So now you know my plan
I bet you think I am crazy
But actually I've done it
'cause my family is lazy

It will save them time and money
If it's planned all well ahead
So they can spend time decluttering
My wardrobe and junk instead!

There is nothing more rewarding than knowing that for once you have got one up on people and have scuppered whatever plans they had for after your demise. This is catharsis at its best and something I mean to take forward in my life. Yes there is absolutely nothing better than for once doing something better than others and if I can't get a bit of self-care smugness from something like arranging my own funeral then when can I? I shall be sat in the hot coals of hell or wherever I end up as a non-believer with a big smirk all over my face. Anyone care to join me?

Self-care whilst gardening

I say I like gardening, but without beating around the bush (pardon the pun) what that means is that it allows me to escape from the house and pulling out weeds helps me see instant success. For me it is the same as decluttering a cupboard indoors. Due to the limited control over my caring role, I need to have some control and deciding which plants to half hack to death and which ones can be gently pruned is entirely up to me. My grandma used to be an amazing gardener and she was known for having the so called 'Green Fingers'. I on the other hand use her name to allow me to get away with cutting back fiercely on the shrubs that need a gentle haircut and I thank her for my 'Green Fingers' when I get it right.

You will be interested to learn that I currently have a greenhouse in complete state of disrepair at the back of the garden by a fence that separates us from the local public house. Sadly their beer garden is the other side of the fence and I initially lost a great deal of glass panes due to footballs and other objects being lobbed or kicked into the trees either on purpose or by mistake. I did on one occasion find a beautiful dice that someone had handmade out of a metal. Goodness knows where I have put that. I also found children's shoes and kindly lobbed them back over the fence. But for now I have a dilapidated greenhouse, overgrown with brambles and full of broken glass and shredded footballs from having come through the glass. I have explained to Andrew that unless the greenhouse is moved then I cannot use it. This is rather stating the obvious as unless I wore armour head to toe and used long handled cutting gear, I was very unlikely to be able to get anywhere close to it.

In order to help me relax, Andrew thought we should sort out the garden. Rather a lot of money later, when I nearly had another cardiac event at the till point due to the cost, it occurred to me that it would be me who would be expected to dig all the shrubs in and it amounted to a total of 40. Now, not saying I am lazy, I like gardening, but digging holes for 40 plants is not the part of gardening I enjoy. I enjoy pulling out the occasional weed, pruning or rather hacking the shrubs and then letting Andrew lug and hump the garden waste to the local tip. I do not in any way shape or form enjoy digging 40 holes, prepping the soil and carefully teasing the roots out etc. That part of gardening is boring, hard work and not a part of the gardening I relish being forced to do.

So, let us have a think about who found themselves digging holes in the garden during Storm Freya and getting soaked to the skin each time it decided to pelt it down with rain. Funnily enough it wasn't Andrew as Andrew had kindly said he would give me a day to relax whilst he took care of Hedge. Hmm,

I am not too sure about relaxing as the next day I woke up completely stiff and aching.

However, on a positive, I did manage some self-care whilst digging as each time I trod the spade into the soil, I swore silently in my head at all the things that were going wrong regarding Hedge's care. It became like a mantra whilst I dug away at the ground and I did power through the 35 holes quicker than I thought. Yes, I know it was meant to be 40 holes, but if you had seen the size of the pots you would appreciate why I had saved the last few for Andrew to dig. Surely that wouldn't be too much to ask. Although I was more than mildly annoyed with Andrew when he quickly mentioned that he might get someone in to dig the last five holes as he was not a digger. Therefore, I can declare that through means of deduction I am a digger, as I dug the last 35 holes. Ok so they were significantly smaller but it was 35 holes all the same.

My next tiny bit of self-care came once I had come back indoors and had a hot shower, followed by some bonding time with Little sis, who had decided it would be nice to play hairdressers with my hair whilst we snuggled to watch a Disney film together. I love having my hair done, so enjoyed most of it, until I realised she had tied it up in tight little braids. My newly acquired mantra was coming into its own when Andrew was attempting to remove the tight bands that held the braids in place. At least I learnt something towards my self-care whilst gardening, a mantra to silently swearing. So if I now appear in deep thought or miles away you will know what I am doing.

Pull up the weeds
And hack the heads
Clear out well
Your flower beds

Sink that spade
With heavy boot
Bury your anger
With each planted root

Cut back shrubs
Let your anger go
Start to feel
Your happiness grow

Silently say a mantra
Let out every sigh
'cause once done
You'll be on a high

Your little bit of self-care
Will have been achieved
So sit and enjoy yourself
Happy and relieved!

Hmm, muddy boots, muddy clothes, a muddy cat from walking through and rolling in the mud (cheers, Borry) and muddy kitchen floor from the muddy cat and muddy child who took off muddy boots but had somehow got mud in her boots and got mud all over the towel after she washed her hands. Oh and muddy duvet cover from the muddy cat. How the heck did the muddy cat go from one end of the house, up the carpeted stairs and still have mud on him? Thanks, Storm Freya, for the mud. I have now forgotten about my self-care and am now washing mud from everything! My digging mantra has now turned into one that also has its uses when scrubbing mud.

More recently I have made up a little song that I sing to irritate the heck out of anyone close by, namely Little sis and Andrew, who are also now not impressed as they have an irritating little song and tune in their heads that they can't get rid of. Here goes…

> I shall dance with the daffodils all day long
> I'll dance with the daisies on the lawn
> I will dance with the bumble bees flower to flower
> And dance with you 'til dawn
>
> I never shall be lonely
> I never shall be sad
> 'cause when I'm by your side
> I'm only ever glad ohhhh I will dance with the daffodils …

> And when the storm clouds gather
> And I am feeling low
> I will always find you
> No matter where you go ohhhh I will dance with the daffodils...

This little song also gets rid of anyone who interrupts me in the garden, so I am left to get on with chopping back anything in my path.

Brexit

I voted to leave the European Union (EU). I like to think of a change is as good as a rest. I remember the day of the vote in great detail as it was the day I got admitted to hospital following a cardiac event I had whilst I was visiting Hedge in hospital. I was attempting to sleep on a busy admissions ward and was roused by the porters coming in moaning loudly that we were to leave the EU and how it would mean a war etc. I soon (like thousands of others) became in simple terms 'done in' when hearing and seeing about it on the TV and became particularly irritated when politicians kept saying they knew that the likes of me didn't mean to leave. Actually my view never changed, I am a stubborn person by nature and I would far rather just have got on with what was promised than keep hearing people argue over it and have the press make news about the leavers and remainers arguing the point. In fact, my self-care was to stop watching the news as it was driving me potty to hear of the constant spin and stories being dug up to discuss.

> Brexit for breakfast, dinner and tea
> Brexit discussed so angrily
> Brexit going on and around in my head
> I wish oh I wish they'd discuss care needs instead

Count up the hours and cost of each MP
Discussing Brexit for breakfast, dinner and tea
I don't want to think, I dare not to comment
'cause I am not sure MPs think what they've spent

Yep I am fed up even considering watching the news
And listening to MPs saying they know the public views
Well actually they don't know mine not even one bit
As I am sick and tired of hearing of it!

Under freedom of information can I make a request?
Can I ask for the costing of MPs when they protest?
Stop the waffle, promises and spin
Either we are out... or we are in!

So, with all the talk of a re-vote and the ranting and raving going on it ended up appearing that the democratic will of the people was no longer valid. Therefore I came up with the nice idea of maybe rewriting a bit of history and re-voting on these events. Who knows, the idea I had may also be the ideas of many. I believe one such example could be to please re-vote the year on 'Britain's Got Talent' when lots of viewers felt that Susan Boyle should have won, I really love her voice. In fact, I love all of her; she is so inspirational. I would also like to re-vote for the Great British Bake Off as I am never keen on who wins each week and feel it should be someone else. Whilst I am at it my mother wrongly voted for a party to represent her at the last local elections and realised once she got home that she had put a cross in the wrong box as she didn't have her reading glasses with her. Can she have her voting paper back again please so she can do it properly next time?

I am enjoying the idea of all these second chances. I also constantly pick the wrong raffle ticket number, so could I have the winning one please? Lastly, next time the draws are done on who plays who at football for the World Cup can we just keep going until the men's England team picks a team which means they will actually get through to the finals and win? Now wouldn't that be great! Oh dear, it really could leave us in a terrible pickle, couldn't it, but quite entertaining. I suspect I am not the only one to be thinking this way! Maybe sarcasm has a place in self-care after all.

College dreams and losses

We had hoped that Hedge would be able to attend college once he was old enough to leave school, but the dire way the mental health services had failed Hedge, meant that was put in the balance. Not to mention the fact that in order to transition to adult services it meant a complete bun fight to decide who would fund what. All this piled on more stress for Hedge and resulted in further deterioration in his mental health. Then just to add in a dollop of more stress, one of the key staff for Hedge left under a cloud. Despite the fact that I implicitly expressed to the staff (I have employed) that whilst I employed staff, I did not hold the budget, nor compose the letters or make the ultimate decision as I had to follow the rules and had my hands tied firmly behind my back, I still got blamed. Unfortunately for this particular member of staff it was simply not possible to offer her the conditions she wanted, due to not being in a position to be able to give everyone the favourable conditions she asked for. If I had offered one member of staff better terms and conditions it would have left me exposed in the eyes of employment law and would have enabled other carers to legitimately request the same conditions due to the precedence being set. This was and still is the downside of managing a Personal Health Budget and one side of life I could seriously have done without. Staff consistently appeared to quickly forget that I had to do as I was told by those who provide the funding and that letters and guidance came and continues to come from the insurance company who dictate how I have to formulate and respond to them. I remain the unpaid middle-man or should I say woman to be politically correct. The time and energy managing the HR (Human Resources) for the carers I employed and continue to employ is ridiculous and certainly not appreciated by those high up who dictate where and how Personal Health Budgets are provided.

So off with a bang went one of our most critical carers. I was devastated that it ended this way after knowing the person for 10 years and the added stress due to the way she took the news certainly took its toll on me and maybe this is what she was hoping for? Sadly I had to spend many hours on the insurance legal line managing her letters of complaint and even set up a hearing to listen to her concerns. Time was taken off work for the hearing which ended up all in vain as she failed to show at the last minute. It saddens me to think that she left the way she did. Her departure from the care team had a markedly negative effect on Hedge and left us all reeling from the aftermath of what had occurred. What makes it worse is that I had purposely recruited knowing the characters I had in the team and on one occasion she had pointedly told me she would leave if I so much as interviewed a person she had previously known. All I know is that I always protected my staff as much as I could, but all too quickly their loyalties would change when it suited. Not saying this was the case with this particular carer, but many have left feeling that I have somehow crossed them. If only they knew how much I spoke out for them and championed their corner when discussing their roles and abilities.

I yet again had another one of my depleted team leave and this also ended up as a sour note in the end. I like to think that it may be the carer's way of trying not to feel guilty when they leave due to the situation they put myself and Hedge in. All I hope for is that others do not keep promising the earth when they have absolutely no intention of keeping to their promises. Having said we would have the care agency step up if and when any of our own carers left meant that transferring more to care agency staff was happening quicker than we anticipated. However, the care agency like ourselves, were also struggling to recruit due to the problem of there being a recruitment crisis due to not enough carers applying for caring roles. I surmise this is the same old problem throughout the country as there is still only the same carer pool to recruit from.

Therefore, College was put on hold and the Educational Healthcare Plan went into the ether and vanished with no meeting, no letters, no nothing. Not even an acknowledgement that it was ceasing and so there became a huge void for Hedge to fill. Nevertheless it meant I could declutter the old school room as it would no longer be needed. Maybe this was my self-care positive, that at last I had one tidy decluttered room. Ok so I am forgetting about the other small irritation like the fact I have now got Hedge going on and on that he has lost his college place, but let me tell you through slightly gritted teeth that I now have a decluttered room.

Being an appointee to Personal Independence Payments (PIPs)

Predictably there was no other appropriate choice, but me, to be Hedge's appointee. Hedge is dire with money, no doubt like a lot of others his age. Understandably I can't help thinking back to when I was 19 years old, driving a car, going out to nightclubs, letter boxing on the moors and holding down a full-time job and part-time job. I was fortunate enough to not have had a disability that was constantly holding me back. Nevertheless, I still managed to save money and appreciate its worth as I was on a strict budget if I went out with my friends. As for Hedge he has no true understanding for the value of money and I can't blame him for that. We knew Hedge had dyscalculia; however, school failed to test him due to Hedge either being unwell on the day of the test or the person who was meant to be completing the test leaving. This challenge with numbers has left Hedge unable to understand the basics. Hedge knows I hold his money for him, but that I do give him the money when he asks and wearingly he asks me most days. At the end of one month Hedge had spent so much on buying and selling that I explained to him that like me he would have to be poor until the end of the month as I had also overspent at the beginning. Hedge thinks of everything as a bargain, but has no concept of just how much it costs to live. If you can't do sums and don't understand sequencing, why would you understand how long money needs to last and what it is to be spent on?

The fun and games of being the appointee means that it is solely down to me to let the PIPs people know the moment Hedge is admitted to hospital and then down to me to let them know he is home again. Sounds straightforward, doesn't it? Unless like me you also have the pleasure of being an appointee so know how frustrating the whole process is! Sadly, it is never that simple. I have now learnt to put the phone on loud speaker whilst I have a coffee and allow myself time to have an hour to read a magazine (usually somewhat out of date as it is my only opportunity to read like this). However much I try to ignore the irritating classical music that is being played on a never ending circuit, the music remains in my brain for the rest of the day. On the plus side I do get to practise self-care whilst drinking a cup of hot coffee. See, it is amazing when and where you can actually grab a nearly relaxing bit of time to relax!

Then the call handler requests a million and one security questions so it feels more like an interrogation before you can tell them that your child (who you are appointee for) is back in hospital.

I did have one laugh out loud time when phoning in to advise the call handler that Hedge was now out of hospital. The call handler answered the phone and asked for the date the person was released from prison. Whilst I liken the stays in hospital to prison only a damn sight more costly because you have to pay for the TV and I understand it is all free in prison, surely the call handler could have got his stock reply correct. I also have to pay for parking and put up with a bay full of other people butting in on my conversations, alongside having to listen to them decide they need a commode part way through a meal. I can only think being in prison might be slightly better as at least no one is sitting on a commode (while they try to ignore the odour or sounds of flatulence) whilst they are eating their meal and the TV is free. I imagine sleeping at night might be slightly better in prison too, although I am only basing my knowledge on watching the reruns of 'Porridge'.

Anyhow back to the call handler who embarrassingly apologised and I burst out laughing in near hysteria after having waited almost an hour for him to pick up. The poor man was mortified, but I politely told him it had made my day as I needed a laugh. So there we have it, yet another bit of self-care and this time when I least expected it, as I was still chuckling to myself hours later!

On the negative side I had hoped that someone else could pretend to be me on the phone as if I am at work or stuck in hospital it is not possible for me alone to spend almost an hour on the phone waiting for someone to pick up. However, I am told it has to be me.

Grab self-care where you can
A little here and there
Let your self-care happen
Anytime and anywhere

Grab a coffee, or cup of tea
Sneak a biscuit in
Whilst waiting on the phone
It really is win-win!

Let the classical music
Help you modify
Read that magazine
It's either laugh or cry

Take each and every moment
Try being flirty on the phone
It's far better being happy
Than boring and alone

Once the call is over
It's one less job to do
Tick it off your list
Be proud of being you!

Another such delight as appointee was giving Hedge the £50.00 he needed to collect his laptop from the computer repair shop. I had explained to Hedge on many occasions that I already paid insurance for the laptop which would have meant it being repaired for free. Infuriatingly I could have just reset the laptop to an earlier time and it would have got rid of the so-called virus. It was easy money for the repair shop and sadly has now voided the insurance. Goodness knows why Hedge decided to take the laptop to the repair shop (with his carer). The trouble is, Hedge has memory problems so unless the carers listen to what I explain to them then Hedge has no hope in managing his money any better.

If only I had £50.00 to waste like this then I would be very happy. It is with pleasure that I can now say I am now very happy. The hospital where I work has started giving free parking, so instead of feeding the meter I put the money in my purse and saved up £50.00 to spend as I please. I told Andrew and Little sis that I would treat us all to a meal out. What was even better was the fact that when I came to pay at the restaurant they said they no longer took cash, so I was forced to pay on the credit card. My self-care just keeps getting better by the moment. The credit card is a joint one with Andrew and I very rarely end up putting anything towards the final payment. So I still have £50.00 in change to spend on anything I like. I was endeavouring not to smile too much when Andrew queried how he thought I was treating us to a meal out. My reply: "I have treated you to the idea, the good company and the enjoyment of the food, it's not my fault they no longer take cash." I am so loving the new self-care spirit for life that I am getting into.

Mug embossed across my forehead

Being a carer, I frequently feel I have 'mug' embossed across my forehead. It was fantastic that after many years of trying I succeeded in getting my carer's assessment completed, but in all reality what did it provide? I very kindly got allocated some funding to enjoy myself, but without carers to take over when exactly was I meant to do what I wanted to do? When I was not at work, I got the strong sense of glee oozing from the lips of those who were having difficulty recruiting. It was assumed by all and sundry that because I was at home then I would care for Hedge. I love Hedge dearly but being forced into training the carers from an agency was not exactly what I had in mind when we decided to no longer recruit carers via Direct Payments. I was exhausted from not being able to do what I wanted and escape the life I found myself bound to. The agency managers we were dealing with were lovely, but as they did not have anything to say about recruitment, it was taking longer and longer to train staff who did not have enough experience to look after Hedge. My staff did approximately 4 - 6 shadow shifts, whereas the agency was requiring up to 14 + shadow shifts. I therefore had to put my foot down and said enough is enough and that I would not be training staff more than a couple of induction shifts and the rest would be up to them. It was not for me to keep telling people what was expected of them when they worked; the agency would have to take some responsibility.

Therefore, rather than keep bemoaning how exhausted I was, I stuck to my guns and told everyone that I was unavailable for a few days in order for us to take Little sis to an 'Over The Wall' siblings camp. The organisation is a charity that offers free residential activity camps in medically safe environments for children with serious illnesses and separate camps for their siblings -- empowering children to be children. This excuse of dropping off and picking up Little sis conveniently doubled up as providing desperately needed head space. It niggled me then and continues to niggle me how Hedge's carers moaned when they had to work more than a few shifts together. Gallingly I can't leave, I am stuck and so is Hedge and "muggins" in other words "me" will keep getting called upon unless I made a selfish stand and say "No, I will not be here".

> Mug sums up quite a bit
> When I think of the caring role
> It means carer without a choice
> That kind big hearted soul
>
> Mug is the way I feel
> When I try to object

Then I do it anyway
To avoid accusations of neglect

Mug comes in many guises
Yet to me it gives no voice
I get on with my caring role
Neither option nor no choice

For me this 'mug' is tired
She wants a life of her own
Yet no-one really wants to know
This 'mug' feels so alone

So the 'mug' will carry on
Giving free care at a cost
'cause due to my dedication
My freedom and life is lost

'Mug' is what I am
Not what I want to be
As all the time I am there
The others fail to see

'Mug' will do the caring
'Mug' will train the staff
'Mug' will be exhausted
'Mug' will cry or laugh

'Mug' is not a word
That the Government use
To describe all the carers
That they don't pay and abuse

I am a proud mother 'mug'
A tad grumpy and grey
Needing 'me time' not guilt
And some self-care today!

Andrew took time off work and the both of us enjoyed the long drive there and back and we treated ourselves to lunch in a pub. The journey provided the self-care time we craved and seeing the look of excitement on the face of Little sis when she arrived at camp made it all the more worthwhile. Little sis could be Little sis with other young carers without coming second best all the time and we for once were not feeling guilty that she had missed out yet again due to a sudden cancellation of a break away due to her big brother being hospitalised. I won't deny that I shed a tear in the car as we dropped her off. Not a tear that I was about to miss Little sis, but one of relief that finally Little sis got some attention and fun all to herself and this time no emergency dashes to hospital could ruin her fun. So, thank you 'Over The Wall' for providing me and thousands of other families the space to recuperate and recharge our batteries and for providing children with the opportunity to be children.

Technology and self-care

Andrew went to Dubai for two weeks. Andrew reckoned he was going to have a hard time getting through the two weeks and felt that he would rather be at home. As for me, I would rather be in Dubai. Andrew may have been working but I was once again bottle green with envy about the fact that in the evenings he would get to do what he wants due to no-one being a burden on him. Burden may sound a strong word to some and yes I do love Hedge and Little sis. Note the hint of sarcasm, but my caring life is burdened like a donkey taking a heavy load and being forced to plod on regardless of how exhausted I feel. Maybe I was a donkey in my last life, as I am sure I will just drop dead one day, and people will turn their heads and not even contemplate why it happened to someone so young. Ok maybe not quite so young now, I like to dream.

Now back to Dubai, dearest Andrew (said by myself through gritted teeth) had downloaded WhatsApp on his mobile. There was nothing wrong with that other than I usually prefer to go hands-free and carry on doing the housework, feed the cat, sit on the toilet, brush my teeth, put the bins out and generally get on with things when I am on the phone. Now I was forced to sit trying to adjust the phone so that I didn't look like Les

Dawson in drag, modelling an added double chin. I am all for modern technology but it was not helping my self-care one bit. Fortunately when Andrew phoned my wrinkles didn't appear to be too noticeable or the fact that my hair urgently needed washing. I won't be disingenuous and pretend to know how the younger generation get on using WhatsApp or Messenger for phone calls. I fell in love dreaming of the man behind Andrew's voice and oddly enough seeing him semi-reclined in bed showing me more of his left nostril than I would like due to his weirdly angled head is ruining all my fondest memories of him. So instead of chillaxing in my favourite comfy PJs I was sat trying to adjust the screen to make me look like the super model I would like to be. Goodness knows what I must have looked like in the full picture; it was bad enough seeing the tiny square of me in one corner of the phone.

So as for self-care and having a quick slurp of coffee, I couldn't as WhatsApp failed miserably to enhance my looks and the last time I did slurp coffee whilst using WhatsApp, I managed to slurp coffee down my chin and onto my top. Not quite the sexy older woman look I was hoping for.

Years ago, when Andrew worked in Germany, I sent him a letter each day and we spoke on the phone once a month. Absence made my heart grow fonder in those days due to my imagination. Now I had nothing to imagine, I could even view him plodding around in his short sleeved PJs that I had packed for him. All I can say is that I am grateful I met Andrew in the

TECHNOLOGY AND SELF-CARE

days before WhatsApp, as I know for sure that we would not be together now if we had used WhatsApp. I would have soon grown tired of tarting myself up to look good and he would probably have noticed that I have a wonky smile. I am not anything like Olivia Newton-John who Andrew had a teenage crush on, more shall I put it Danny DeVito or Les Dawson as mentioned earlier. Without a doubt I would recommend steering clear of WhatsApp and Messenger unless you look amazing in photos. Otherwise just play a game on your phone instead. Little sis tried to get me to do a word search game on my phone one evening and I apparently didn't even have the brain of a tadpole, so I have a feeling I'll stick to playing Pet Rescue instead!

Technology and self-care
It doesn't help me at all
I've tried and given up
It makes me look a fool

WhatsApp is great
If you've no double chin
I've tried different angles
But I really can't win

I look like a suet pud
When I see the screen of me
I dread to think what Andrew thinks
From what he can see

As for the word games
I have no hope at all
I got told I had a tadpole brain
It drove me up the wall

So I will ignore the technology
Self-care will have to wait
'cause if I use technology
I'll end up in a state!

Sleep

I had always assumed that sleep would be better once my children were older, but actually it has deteriorated. The reason why is that I seem to have more to do before going to bed. Andrew just goes to bed. I tidy round, call the cat in, put the washing on the airer, wash up, dust, sort out a cupboard, and sort the post and so on. Then once in bed I have to pretend I can't hear Andrew snoring. I then find myself getting more and more stressed to the point where murder enters my mind. I have been known to record Andrew snoring and play it back full blast to wake him up. So in order to soothe my nerves I relax in bed and have a snippet of self-care playing 'Pet Rescue' until I am too tired to care about the snoring and fall asleep. I can avoid reality, bury my head in the sand and rescue a cute pet, even if I can't rescue Hedge from the dire situation he is in.

As for Hedge his sleep is all over the place. When I have to care for him due to a breakdown in care cover, I keep my fingers crossed that he will lie in, otherwise he is full on. I am in dire need of a lie in. I consider a lie in to be 7am now, but I would without hesitation like to stay in bed until 9am for just one day without being woken up by either the carer telling me the next carer has failed to show or Hedge ringing me about something insignificant. If I turn my phone off, then the landline rings and that is worse as I have to get out of bed to go and get the phone, only to find that it is Hedge or a cold caller trying to sell me something. I really can't win.

I have on the rare occasion just gone to bed for a lie down due to having a bad headache and reappeared for no-one to realise I was gone, but to only ask what is for dinner. No-one notices if I am not feeling great and I might need to take to my bed, even if I am rustling the box of Paracetamols trying to give a hint.

I think I am fast becoming a hypochondriac. I recently convinced myself I had deteriorating eyesight only to realise it was my daft energy saving light bulbs that makes the whole room appear dimly lit. Whilst on the subject of eyes I almost made an appointment for my eyes to be checked due to flashing lights. On this occasion I can see how I made the mistake. I had got up one dark morning, put on my energy saving light which remained dim whilst I fiddled around looking for my eyeliner. The eyeliner I had put on was called Twilight. Twilight was given as the name for a particular reason as it contains a bit of silver glittery stuff in it. The flashing lights were purely due to my eyeliner catching the light when I blinked. The eyeliner was an old one I used to use on nights out. I really do either need a night out, a sleep in or to sort out my makeup bag. Whichever way it is, I need more sleep to stop making me feel so damned paranoid about my eyesight.

Sleep is a privilege
I get it where I can
But if the snoring is loud
I'm really not a fan

Some days I just plod on
I rest my head anywhere
It may be by a hospital bed
Or comfy reclining chair

Paid carers get a break
To rest their weary eyes
For me there is no escape
No-one hears my sighs

Just let me slumber on
Don't loudly ask if I'm OK
I need to rest my head
So take heed of what I say

My self-care of sleep
Is needed for today
A little nap here and there
Will keep the Zs at bay!

Self-care and sleeping peacefully – don't even get me started. I have learnt to play dead if the cat decides to leap across the bed, I have learnt to play dead if the doorbell rings, I have learnt to play dead if the phone rings, I have learnt to play dead – yes I wish I hadn't learnt to play dead when Andrew forgot I was playing dead and invited the Chippy (Carpenter) to look at the door hinges. Sometimes, just sometimes I could happily do a group scream alongside all the other carers out there. So instead I play dead ignoring the embarrassment of the poor Chippy as he nips quickly back around the door and say a cheery "morning," when I go downstairs for that first cup of coffee.

Even having experienced this mortifyingly embarrassing situation I would still endorse the art of playing dead. If memory serves me correctly I also did a good playing dead act when I was staying at Andrew's parents' bungalow when they were away on holiday. The last thing I expected was the window cleaner to pop through the garden gate. I was rather shy in those days and must have looked incredibly sunburnt as my poor face was feeling very hot and bothered. I did manage to discreetly turn over and was cursing at how long he was taking. I am relieved to say it is a skill that I have now performed to perfection!

Computer use

Hedge's idea of safe internet use is non-existent. A children's Social Worker (prior to Hedge becoming an adult) told Hedge that he should get a Facebook account and another professional told him he should join a dating site. Quite why both of these professionals said what they did remains a mystery. Hedge has no ability to vet people who make contact, thinks of everyone as his friend and has had some incredibly nasty fallings out due to things he has typed that he would never have said out loud. I am sure this rings true with many parents/carers without additional needs. Nevertheless, Hedge is extremely vulnerable as he lacks the ability to weigh up situations and is far from streetwise. Hedge is also not capable of getting the hint that someone is getting fed up due to his constant messaging and he then gets really upset and offended when they block him.

I am sometimes proud of what Hedge posts as he has posted some really thoughtful comments. Disappointingly there have been numerous fallings out with family members over posting private photographs that they would prefer not to be shared online for the world to see and even when they tell him, Hedge will not fully appreciate the impact on that person. This can then end up in a many-hours' conversation going over and over and over the same issue, until I feel completely drained.

Hedge emailed saying I was being unreasonable for wanting him to change his security settings on Facebook so I emailed him back the following poem.

Dearest 'The Hedge'

Facebook is not an excuse
For being safe and sound
It often leads to trouble
When gossip goes around

It often leads to anger
It often leads to stress
The stress just becomes addiction
When friends requests grow less

Don't rely upon the promises
Don't expect people to be honest too
As sadly being honest is something
People on Facebook rarely do

They brag about their lives
They make out they are the best
When really they're no more than me or you
Believe me this is not something that I jest

So be sensible with your friend requests
Be honest, don't be so keen to make
Or be so desperate for a Facebook friend
That you make a big mistake

If ever anyone asks for your password
Tell them no and don't give in
Or your credibility will soon be heading
For the Facebook friendship bin

Trust me that I know
I've had training on the dangers
That so-called friend requests
Are often dodgy strangers

Keep safe and well, seek out
The honest non-judgemental ones
Who can keep you safe on the net
My handsome happy son!

More to the point through practising self-care when looking after Hedge, I positively encourage Hedge's use of the internet. It allows me to take five minutes out to enjoy a cup of coffee, knowing all too well that I will be dealing with the fall-out after I have taken my last slurp of caffeine. I always tell Hedge that when I need a coffee he needs to let me have it in peace and quiet otherwise I might get grumpy. It is one of my rules that

'THE UNOFFICIAL SELF-CARE GUIDE FOR CARERS'

I need to insist upon. This allows me some time to collect my thoughts before I have to continue listening to and answering the barrage of questions I get after I have put my cup down for the final time. Therefore the words "drinking, still drinking, swallowing, breathing, still drinking," are now used on a daily basis in order to provide me with a snippet of self-care time.

Bargain hunting

The internet is also used to surf for bargains, whether it is old board games, old gaming machines or just any old junk that Hedge has decided he desperately needs. The most recent purchase from an online site was a set of old board games. I am sure the lady who sold them must have been delighted, as it saved her bin from getting too full. The carer had no choice but to take Hedge to the house to collect them and did try to discourage the sale. However, Hedge is very persistent and as I have often said 'a bad choice is not necessarily the wrong choice'. Only most of us learn from our mistakes and see consequences to our actions and learn to not do the same thing again. Clearly Hedge does not learn from his mistakes or see consequences. So back to the board games, most of the games had lids so sticky taped together that it was remarkable they did still fit together and the contents were either partially torn or missing. I then had the trip to the local charity shop to dispose of the not so bad games that he already had and binned the others.

Being mindful of never missing an opportunity for self-care, I grabbed this wasted bit of my free time and browsed the books in the charity shop and found myself a lovely book on palmistry. From what I can tell I will never be a palm reader and I am not about to be famous. I then picked up something even better in the local stationery shop next door, which was a fortune-telling ball. I am now using this to give answers to Hedge's many questions. The fortune-telling ball appears to keep both Hedge and Little sis entertained. However, I doubt this will mean that I will run a cattery with Hedge, like the fortune-telling ball kindly told Hedge was 'Possible' after he asked for its opinion on that idea.

Maybe I should make my own fortune-telling bag where Hedge can pick out answers that I have placed in there already that say words on like 'I agree your mum is right', 'Listen to what you are told', 'Don't keep asking so many questions'. The list is endless; I could have a great bit of self-care doing that!

Bargains on the internet
It totally buys me in
If I bid on eBay
I could outbid and win!

The selling sites are fab
With bargains galore
Who knows what I might buy
When I knock upon their door

It will stop me being bored
When I surf and get a deal

BARGAIN HUNTING

I really need it all
The junk is such a steal

I'll fill my house with items
Randomly bought and claimed
More for Mum to moan about
She says I should be ashamed

I've wasted so much money
And half of it is broken
But I've had my fun
My adult voice has spoken

I can waste my money
Bills are sorted by my mum
I can keep ordering on the internet
Whilst I sit upon my bum

Mum can nag and worry
Whilst all I do is buy
I am an adult now
I don't need to justify!

Only I didn't quite appreciate
That money is needed for bills
That debit cards use money
When I pay for food at tills

> I don't understand my finance
> Or even how to forward plan
> But what the heck just spend
> As I am now a full grown man!

Sad isn't it how just because one day you turn from 17 to 18 years old, that young person is suddenly meant to be capable of managing their money. I have tried many systems in order to give some independence and have learnt to relax over items wrongly bought. I have learnt to acknowledge that if Hedge was an able bodied 19 year old he might be at the pub downing beer and wasting money that way, so instead if he wants to waste money on useless items then that is up to him. Another great self-care tip to me is to find better things to worry about than a few old board games that some random lady charged money for. At least Hedge has evidence of his spending, other than a hangover from an alcoholic drink at a pub.

Embarrassing moments whilst attempting self-care

I will do almost anything to grab a few minutes and like many parents hide in the bathroom pretending to need the toilet to just escape for a few minutes. However, on one occasion I was sat on the chair in the bathroom giving my head some very needed space, when my mobile phone started ringing in my pocket. I answered and it was Hedge rambling on about something that I was really not wanting to start going over again, so I patiently explained I was in the toilet. I had just put the phone down when it rang again and Hedge was grilling me once again. Again, I put the phone down after having explained I was in the toilet. By now I was wondering if my plan of escape was giving me the few minutes' break I needed.

I like to think that I am one step ahead so I took a photo of the bathroom in order to reinforce where I was and pinged it off with a message saying 'I am stuck in the toilet'. Only much to my horror realised that I had texted the photo to my father instead. Seconds later I got a message back from my father who lives six miles away to ask if he needed to come over to help me get out of the toilet and who would have a key. I then

'THE UNOFFICIAL SELF-CARE GUIDE FOR CARERS'

phoned my father and told him that it was all a mistake and I had only sent the text to try and stop Hedge keep pestering me. Sadly my sniggering at the whole situation brought Hedge to the outside of the toilet door, where he was banging loudly to get my attention and the door flung open as he had managed to break the lock (part of the door frame and lock to be precise). So the morale of this short story is don't pretend you are in the toilet unless you can be quiet enough to justify that you are parked on the toilet and don't bother texting photographs of where you are unless you can be certain that you are sending them to the correct person! The whole toilet-gate affair ended up costing me a small fortune as I had to pay for a carpenter to sort the door frame and put a new lock on the door for me. It was a costly mistake that I will now be careful not to repeat, hence me pre-warning others of what not to do in an attempt for a bit of self-care.

> Give me just five minutes
> Even a second on the loo
> I need a little break
> Just a minute or two
>
> I need to hide
> To sit and think
> Although in preference
> I'd rather have a drink

EMBARRASSING MOMENTS WHILST ATTEMPTING SELF-CARE

Don't sit outside
Or start to call
I need five minutes
That's 'my rule'

No banging on the door
Just leave me alone
I'll speak when I'm out
You don't need to phone

If you don't believe
I'll even flush the loo
That way you'll never guess
Or even have a clue

Just let me chill
And have my break
I need self-care time
Oh for goodness sake! (through gritted teeth)

A day off to attempt self-care

Fantastic, finally a day off where I could do what I wanted and maybe catch up a bit, maybe going through my trillions of junk emails, potter around and drink caffeine all day. The day started abruptly due to the cat waking me up with his running dive at my head as he scooted across the pillows and then swiping the alarm clock onto the floor. He then proceeded to claw at a magazine on the bedroom floor, undoubtedly thinking I was going to believe he needs to go outside to relieve himself. Fortunately I am not easily fooled as I have watched him do this before when I have been mug enough to get up and let him out and he just saunters out the door and sits and washes his face in the sunshine. Therefore I throw a pillow in his direction and he just sits there winking at me with his big green eyes before jumping up on the bed on top of me and proceeding to fall asleep. Ok so I am now awake, thanks cat! I am being completely crushed by a hefty Borry of 8+ Kgs. So I shove the annoying, now loudly purring cat off me and get up for the day. I then have three delicious Lancashire Eccles cakes for breakfast and a hot strong coffee, before Little sis appears already in her school uniform. I manage to brush her hair without a murmur. Usually it sounds like I am murdering her as I try to brush her hair, but today she is happy and not shouting out saying I am hurting her. So after a quick breakfast and drop off to school I return back home ready to chillax for the day.

I pop upstairs to check my emails and see one has come through advising me of a policy I have not renewed for my car insurance and asking if I could fill out a questionnaire. My stress levels immediately rise and I feel an instant hot flush coming on and a horrid nauseous feeling, as I realise that I have been driving a car minus valid car insurance. I run back downstairs and go through the last week's unopened post to find a renewal quote addressed to Andrew. I can see how the problem occurred, as Andrew is out of the country and his post was in a pile waiting for him to sort. However, that explanation does not quell my stress levels. Panic levels rising, I grab for the telephone and after waiting for an extremely long 15 minutes, get through to talk to a call handler. I explain the situation and she kindly agrees to renew my policy. I would usually have price matched, but was definitely not in the position to do this, so grudgingly paid up the insurance money. I flick the kettle switch down and am almost about to sit back down when the first of 32 phone calls occurs.

The first of many calls was from Hedge's newest carer and the rest were a combination of him and Hedge phoning me as Hedge was not feeling very well. I could have gone over, but due to the extremely long period of training the carer had received, over and above what anyone else has ever had I needed him to find his own feet and start thinking for himself. I guessed that as Hedge kept phoning me and having a rant that he could not be that ill. Therefore, I gave some instructions over the phone and went out in the car to a local discount store. Whilst in the store I received another five phone calls. I answered but kept saying I am not at home I am out.

Between the phone calls, I did enjoy my browsing and ended up coming out of the shop with two lots of extra strong twisty garden twine, a neck travel pillow and some gardening gloves. Random stuff, but could come in useful! I drop off a bag of bits for the local charity shop and arrive home and then it dawns on me. It is Friday afternoon and I have been acting like it was the beginning of the week when the world still continues until the weekend.

After another four phone calls I run to the chemist to collect medication that a GP has ordered and leg it around to the GP Surgery to query where the medication chart is and for confirmation that someone will be coming from the nursing team to administer the intravenous medication Hedge needs. Much to my horror there has been nothing arranged. I am asked to sit and wait and see a GP who says he thought from his conversation with the carer that the carers would be administering the medication. I wanted to cry and by now my face was flushed a tad red with stress. I politely informed the

GP that I needed the medication chart to be completed and that it was him who had to refer to the nurses, not me. The GP (bless him) began to join me in looking concerned and also started to rise in colour. Believe me I was more pillar box red, than the gentle tinge the GP had gone. Even so the GP and I were well aware of the fact it was already 15:45 hours and a Friday. I departed from the Surgery holding onto the medication chart and promises from the GP to say he would immediately contact the nursing team. I hot footed back home and almost threw the medication and drug chart at the carer and Hedge, before running back into my house to make another quick coffee. Down goes the kettle's switch again. Only I realise the time and it is now time for me to collect Little sis from school to get her to her evening class. On the way there the phone goes another five times. I answer on hands free the ones from the Long Term Conditions Nurse but ignore the others. I felt like screaming. Little sis and I drove to a supermarket, collected a meal deal for Little sis and I treated myself to a bottle of wine and some hot spicy potato wedges. I went on to grab an hour of almost pure indulgence whilst greedily stuffing hot spicy potato wedges into my mouth whilst sitting in the car waiting for Little sis to come out of her evening class. Ok so there was the small issue of trying to open the frustrating plastic packet of BBQ sauce and I did end up having to get my car keys to it, but in the end I did open it, even if it did squirt all over my steering wheel. The effort was worth it and I had some self-care time too. I was still thirsty, but gulped down my second cup of coffee of the day once home. Oh and I did forget to mention that I answered another five phone calls between Hedge and his carer when I was sat eating, but my munching got rid of some of my annoyance towards the pair of them.

Little sis was eventually fast asleep in bed and I readily indulged in a glass or two of wine. I sat there knowing that tomorrow is Saturday and it will start early as I have to take Little sis to two clubs and then spend the rest of the day caring for Hedge as the carer is only booked for part of it. I am not a religious person, but I am now praying to whoever wants to listen, that Hedge is in better form tomorrow, as having to look after Little sis and Hedge is not my idea of fun. Roll on Andrew getting home from his trip abroad. Being emerald green with envy is not a colour that suits me well and it is a colour I am fast growing into.

A day to myself

I've a day to myself
I cannot believe
A full day of pampering
So much to achieve

A gentle start to the day
Coffee and cake
I can dream away big
Clearly my first mistake

A DAY OFF TO ATTEMPT SELF-CARE

I should have guessed
I'd be rushed off my feet
How stupid to think
I'd go shopping for a treat

Life was so much simpler
Without a mobile phone
'cause I used to go out
And be left well alone

Now instead I am hassled
With that damn ringing tone
People just keep bothering me
I wished I'd left it at home

I've collected meds from the pharmacy
Paid a huge bill
Only drunk two coffees
No wonder I am feeling ill

I've gone to see the GP
Taxied Little sis around town
Even got the washing on
Not quite a sit down

I am more tired today
Than ever before

And that's because
I thought self-care was in store!

So my plan is not to plan
Don't expect a day to yourself
'cause it will only disappoint
When your plans stay on the shelf!

Fruity frustrations

Why does it have to be so difficult to get carers to see that buying food and achieving that task is all very admirable, but you do also need to put some effort into creating it into a nourishing meal? You keep hearing the Government health campaigns banging on about healthy eating, but who exactly is monitoring the diets of people who have to rely on carers? Does anyone really care? I am frustrated that carers can come into Hedge's house, happily stick on the oven or microwave to cook their own lunch or tea, but totally ignore the fact that Hedge may possibly be hungry. Hedge does like to eat, he has a soup maker in the house as he loves soup, but only one carer has ever used this and she has now left. It makes me wonder why they just assume they can stick on the oven, microwave, make a cup of tea or coffee and not think about the person who they are looking after and asking first. Would you even go into your parents' home and decide to do all these things without politely asking first? Maybe yes, maybe no, but I know what I would always do. I would also always offer someone else a drink if I was getting one myself. But no, this appears to be rarely the case amongst many of the care agency carers who have supported Hedge in his own home. Or maybe it is just some of Hedge's carers. It drives me to distraction and

I find it quite rude when someone openly goes to get themselves a tea or coffee, but does not offer to make one for me. Is the age of politeness dead?

Anyhow I was yet again pushed into the position of covering the weekend due to no care cover yet again. Yet again I found myself tidying up and breaking down eight large boxes of supplies, because no-one had thought to do this, ordering medications and all the other unappreciated jobs that are crucial to Hedge's care. The final straw came when I went to the fruit bowl to get a banana as I was in need of a healthy nibble and I found highly decomposed fruit of some description in the fruit bowl. Fantastic, so evidently no-one had bothered to look in the bowl. So I ended up having to clean the bowl and left it on the kitchen worktop beside a photo and poem attached in a poly pocket. Sadly I doubted anyone would take the hint that I was not impressed, but hoped the poem would be a more polite way of reminding people what food is being purchased for. When I took the mouldy offending item out of the bowl it went up in a cloud of grey smoke and almost choked me as I accidently inhaled it. Yes you can see I was not impressed.

> I'll have a nice ripe banana
> I'll get one from my bowl
> But what's that all grey and powdery
> That won't help fill my hole

FRUITY FRUSTRATIONS

It's put me off from eating
It might climb out at me
Maybe I'll have an Oreo
To nibble on for my tea

I'm meant to have five a day
But I rarely have even one
No idea who buys this stuff
As it rarely sees the insides of my tum

No point buying fruit
If it decomposes quick
It's like the stuff in the fridge
No wonder I'm feeling sick

I need a proper diet
But if no-one prompts me
I'll forget it being food time
And eat crap again for tea

You use my oven and microwave
To make your own meal
You are here to support me
So what's so hard with that deal?

Just think of me and cook
Don't let the food get thrown out

'THE UNOFFICIAL SELF-CARE GUIDE FOR CARERS'

    Don't sit there eating loads
    Whilst I get offered nowt!

    So OK I do graze
    I nibble quite a bit
    But it can still be healthy grazing
    Healthy nibbles help keep me fit

    I have carers to guide me
    To support me being well cared
    So please just help me
    Mealtimes are nicer if shared!

The self-care tip for this section is don't try and sneak a healthy snack, it simply isn't worth it. I should have stuck to eating another Eccles cake. It would have saved the powdery cloud of grey dust going into my lungs causing me a near coughing fit! Note to self is don't bother trying to be healthy, eat food that you like as it makes you feel good. That is until I start piling on the pounds.

Out of the blue

Having sorted my front garden during the enforced time off work and in between caring for Hedge and attempting to train agency carers, my house was in dire need of a spring clean. So what better way to start the day than to take down the nets, start cleaning the windows and get rid of the cobwebs that have a sneaky way of appearing in the corners of the rooms? Or so I thought...

My mobile phone rang and I picked it up to hear the agency carer asking me if I was available to pop over for a quick chat. I explained that I was in the middle of something, but the desperation in her voice meant that I agreed to pop over for a quick visit. Popping across my front garden and into Hedge's house I immediately detected it was not going to be just a quick chat or visit. Indeed the quick chat and visit ended up being a two day ordeal.

So how did this all occur? By way of explanation the agency, unbeknown to me or Hedge, had employed this particular carer who had a back injury which prevented her from being able to take Hedge out with his mobility scooter. I could see both sides of the story as the carer was a really great carer in every other respect. Unfortunately as Hedge already felt prevented from a 'normal' life due to his disability, being told he could not have choice of where he went on the days that this particular carer worked was in Hedge's terms 'disabling him further not enabling him'. The combination of Hedge's problems processing information, his frustration that yet something else was being denied together with his inability to appreciate I was trying to resolve the situation through purchasing some very expensive car ramps and even contemplating putting the carer on my car insurance (so she could use my car instead) proved too much for Hedge. The world caved in after I had spent an incredibly tense five hours listening and re-explaining the situation. All the while Hedge was becoming more and more distressed and distanced from reality. The resultant adrenalin coursing through Hedge's veins combined frustration and the lack of ability to understand and loss of reality resulted in the police being called. My own brain was fogged and I had been left dazed and exhausted from the mental exertion it took to prevent Hedge suiciding. It is ironic that at the time of the police's arrival, the medical secretary from the Child and Adolescent Mental Health Service (CAMHS) was phoning me to arrange a date for a discharge meeting. The look on the police officer's face was choice when I politely said I needed to answer the phone as it was a hospital number and then told him who was on the line. It is not surprising that the police officer told me that he had come across other situations like this before, where CAMHS were discharging young adults where there was not any service provision available to transition the young person to. I was left wondering whether there was anything I could have done differently, but know in my heart of hearts that the answer to this is a no. However, that annoying inner voice in my head kept casting a doubt on whether I might have been able to do anything different.

The outcome was the police escorting Hedge to the hospital for assessment and me following behind in my car with the wheelchair so that once arriving at the hospital the police could take this off me so that they could book Hedge into the Emergency Department whilst they waited for me to park.

I thought I had grown rhino skin since Hedge was born, but regrettably my rhino skin has not adapted yet to the embarrassment of all the other Emergency Department attendees turning to stare at me when I arrived to take over from the police who were towering above my very slight, agitated son in his wheelchair. The police were amazing, but surely it should not be their role to escort mentally ill patients to hospital due to a lack of mental health services. Mind you, the care and compassion shown by both police officers needs commending as they had far more compassion than many a so-called health professional I have come across and maybe health professionals could learn a thing or two from the police. I am welling up with tears just remembering how relieved I was when they came through the door of Hedge's house, as I don't know how I could have done anything more to prevent a disaster from occurring if the police did not arrive when they did.

Hedge was admitted to hospital on intravenous antibiotics as the doctors felt the altered behaviour was due to an infection. Who knows, what I do know is that Hedge is still being failed and not getting the mental health support he needs. As a result we lost another valued carer as the agency removed her from the package.

To add insult to injury, after having to leave Hedge in the Emergency Department to collect Little sis from her after school club, I had an out of hours Social Worker on the telephone questioning why I had left a vulnerable person alone. Justifiably I was livid at the accusation and I politely reminded her that I was no longer parentally responsible for Hedge as he was now an adult and that I had explained to a nurse that I had to collect my daughter from her after school club and that as she was still a minor, she was my priority. I also reminded the Social Worker that my son was meant to be in a place of safety and that I had not abandoned him. By now I was in serious need of a break and in dire need of throwing my toys out of the pram.

> I look back and wonder
> When did it go wrong?
> Did I over-negotiate?
> Did I wait too long?
>
> I look back and over think
> Should I have given in?

Did I make the situation worse?
And help it all begin

Hedge needs help urgently
We all are sinking fast
Without help will our future
Become Hedge's past?

All we want is help
All Hedge needs is care
Not police escorts to hospital
Whilst people look and stare

I need my son not anxiety
Little sis needs her brother too
But with no support appearing
I doubt this will come true

So in the meantime I'll wait
I will believe in my son
I know he can recover
Because I am his mum!

So in order to practise self-care I bought fish and chips and a treat of mushy peas for tea. Trouble is on this occasion stress meant that I had trouble swallowing the fish and chips as I had a rather annoying stress lump in my throat. The great news was that this annoying lump did not prevent a rather enormous glass of wine from being swigged down in one in order to calm my nerves! So I do not wish anyone reading this to assume there is never any time for self-care as I managed to squeeze in some self-care to help drown my stresses of the day, even if it was a rather unhealthy option. Each chip I stabbed with my fork was jabbed meaningfully and hungrily enjoyed and wine glugged to wash down the chips.

Eccles cakes and friendship

I seem to go through fits and fads of foods, but my favourite is still chips and now added to my rather small list of favourites are real Lancashire Eccles cakes. Oh my goodness don't I kill for an Eccles cake or chips or both. I am sure it is the carbs I am craving due to my body needing comfort food and without any qualms I will happily argue that a carrot stick does not have the same effect. My desire for carbs is huge as is my need for a walk to clear my head. So after eating not one but four Eccles cakes alongside downing a large cup of coffee, I take a wander on my own to support self-care and take a long walk along the quayside. As I walk I realise that in the grand scheme of things I don't count other than counting in my own co-existing world. There are a sea of people also walking, either hand in hand, on their own, walking dogs, pushing buggies and prams and the insignificance of me becomes apparent. As I walk I think and as I think I ponder and as I ponder it dawns on me that unless I look after me, no-one really cares. We are all on our own and it is down to funding, holding onto budgets and the pretence that services care. I am sure that the most conscientious of health professionals cares, but at the end of the day they get to go home and so long as they have safely documented they have done their best they can sleep. It appears to be easier for services to take on people whose needs can be quickly and easily resolved; those who have complex needs like Hedge are failed due to their complexities. Meanwhile the Hedges of this world block up other services and staff can't be released to provide care to others. It is all so wrong, but as a manager of such a service is it better to support the masses or just a few complex cases?

My walk along the quayside ended up with me sat on a bench overlooking the water and in front of me was a boat called 'Friendship'. My friends have stresses that are not dissimilar to my own. Was this a subliminal sign? I very much doubt it, but it did make me smile. Here I am pondering on life and what the few friends I have mean to me when the boat in front of me has the name 'Friendship'. I don't do Facebook with my real name but use a pseudonym and I only have the grand total of 12 friends and I don't count most of them as friends (no criticism meant). As for work, I rarely socialize and put this down to being older. I am married now, have two children and have wisened up to who can be a friend, who is a user and who I can trust in and confide in. This brings me back nicely to my friends whom I can rely on not to judge or chastise me in any way and who take me for who I am. So here's to the boat named 'Friendship'. I have managed self-care with a brisk walk along the quayside and come away appreciating my friends more than ever before. Best of all when I returned back home I enjoyed another Eccles cake.

<blockquote>
Eccles cakes and friendship
What a fine combination
</blockquote>

Knowing both are available
A heart-warming sensation

Cup of coffee in one hand
Eccles cake upon a plate
Phone on loudspeaker
A friend whom to relate

Time to listen
Time to reply
Eccles cake eaten
The minutes soon fly

A weight lifted
A trouble shared
Tears and laughter
Knowing someone has cared

A quick pick me up chat
Just a five minute call
Can add to your self-care
Help you to stand tall

Just don't forget
In good times and bad
It's your non-Facebook friends
Who listen when you're sad

A self-enforced break away

Sometimes it can be extremely hard to stand my ground, but in order to preserve self-care I need to do it every now and then. Like so many other carers I am sure, I have said 'I cannot do this anymore', 'enough is enough', 'I feel like I am going to walk', 'I have reached my limit'. However, I also know that due to the very fact that I am a carer I will continue as I have no choice but to do so, and unless I learnt to mean it when I say no, that this will continue. Therefore I stood my ground and told everyone that I was still going away on a four-day break whilst Andrew was working. This was with the knowledge that Hedge was unwell in hospital and his entire care package had fallen. We were left with a few carers, one of whom was new to care work and although he may have felt he was doing a splendid job, I am sorry to say was woefully inept at the simplest of things. However, having not had a break away for five long years I needed to escape and recoup and get my head around things. This was the very first time that Andrew and myself had been away with absolutely no responsibility whatsoever since before we had Hedge some 20 years ago. We were determined to escape in spite of feeling guilty and having to contend with 'inner feelings' of guilt that we had, as Hedge kindly told us, we had 'abandoned him'. On the positive side Andrew was saving time not commuting as we were staying in our motorhome and we were able to have time together in the evening when he returned 'home' from a day at work.

As luck would have it by day two of the four-day break I was feeling terrible. I had broken out in a head cold and had a muzzy head. I also couldn't quite relax. As a friend who texted me late the previous night mentioned, you can take a horse to water, you can't make it drink. I had taken myself away in order to relax, but I just couldn't quite relax and I was now feeling cooped up unable to do much at all. This was absolutely ridiculous as I was sure that once I was back in the thick of it I would be desperate for time to chill. You just can't win.

I think I needed time for baby steps to relaxation and I should have just taken an afternoon off, not thought about escaping for four days. I doubt I am alone on this one. I was nonetheless having the fun of watching an entire collection of a series on TV that I never got to watch at home.

The moral of my inability to relax is: learn to take small snippets of relaxation, not try to grab huge chunks of time as it can be quite impossible to relax and it might lead to more stress, not less as it did for me.

'THE UNOFFICIAL SELF-CARE GUIDE FOR CARERS'

Relax when you can
Don't wait for a break
As waiting too long
Can be a mistake

Learn to take each moment
Learn to take each day
A little snippet of time
To brush cobwebs away

Don't expect to relax
If you force yourself too
You'll feel guilty like hell
Believe me it's true

You'll sit and procrastinate
Worry and churn
A hole in your heart
Beginning to burn

A greater self-care
Would be better spent
Taking tiny baby steps
Self-care with intent!

Returning from a few days' self-enforced break

I was totally insane to have thought that returning after my break away would put me in a relaxed frame of mind on my return. I returned with a heavy cold still in full flow and an exacerbation of my asthma and feeling guilty that I had abandoned Little sis (not actually abandoned but that is how it felt).

I spent the entire of the first day home emailing, telephoning and speaking to Hedge and different health professionals over the lack of care Hedge had received whilst I had been on my mini-break.

This had not been helped by the care agency suddenly deciding they would not provide care whilst Hedge was in hospital, so were in attendance to babysit rather than ensure that he continued to receive his care needs. The carers had even been given paperwork to sign in agreement with the care agency's new policy. I could happily have screamed, but couldn't as my voice was too sore to scream.

At the time of commissioning the agency, we were told that they could deliver all care, so I was incredibly cross that they had suddenly changed their minds. This change of policy left Hedge vulnerable and once again lacking appropriate support.

During this sudden change of policy by the care agency, there was a failure to refer to the hospital dietician, a failure to deliver care as per Hedge's care plan and more importantly Hedge was feeling terribly let down by the agency that he previously had trust in. It appeared that Hedge has been failed yet again due to inappropriate staff being employed and paid handsomely for just sitting there talking to Hedge.

I lost count of the amount of emails and telephone calls I made and how many different staff I discussed Hedge with. Hedge very much lost faith in the care agency who promised the earth when they took on the care package and managed to spectacularly fail him when he was at his most vulnerable as a patient in hospital. By now I had involved, amongst others, the Safeguarding Team, Complex Discharge Team, the Commissioner and the hospital's own Patient Advice Liaison Service.

I woke yet again with no hope of anything being resolved, but to my surprise an urgent telephone conference had been called between interested parties, with promises to get back to me and update me once they had spoken and gathered all their information. Sadly in the time that all these shenanigans had been going on Hedge's mental health had taken a real bashing once again and he was feeling incredibly let down by everyone.

In the interim the care agency continued to refuse to do anything other than sit in a chair by Hedge and one of the carers decided to put on headphones and listen to music whilst on his phone all day. Hedge stated it would be better to have a shop dummy sat beside him, as he would not have to listen to the thumping music coming from the carer's phone. Hedge and I both agreed on this suggestion of his and how ridiculous the situation had become. We felt united in our confusion as to how the care agency could suddenly change their policy from delivering care in hospital to just sitting there doing nothing. My mother now in her eighties cheekily asked if she could be taken on by the agency as she fancied a change of scene and could easily read a magazine with the added bonus of earning some money. Even Little sis was asking how old she needed to be to be taken on by the agency as she had managed to work out how much she could earn a day for doing nothing and was saving up for art and craft materials and more books. The downside was that if any of us were to be employed by the agency we would also have to listen to Hedge protesting on how he no longer trusted the agency.

Much to my disbelief I had an email from the agency telling me that they have another member of staff ready to be trained. I promptly emailed the care agency and forwarded a copy of the email to the other relevant parties involved (below is an excerpt of the email that has been edited for anonymity):

'I really don't know how anyone is going to be trained if they are not going to be able to do anything per the agency policy. Hedge is currently not very happy with the agency and I very much doubt he will be happy for a new person to just sit with him and do nothing, or indeed have her shadowing another person doing nothing.'

I know for a fact the ward staff were far from happy as they are running around like headless chickens trying to do everything for Hedge whilst a carer was just sat there on their phone listening to music. I can't begin to imagine how the ward staff would feel if two carers were sat there doing nothing, with one carer learning from the other doing nothing.

I truly hoped that something would be resolved as Hedge no longer had confidence in the current agency and his two kittens were due to arrive within the next few weeks. Fortunately as a complete and utter cat lover I wasn't stressed about the kittens, although I was not sure that my old Borry would appreciate the kittens moving in. However, being mindful that it was unlikely that the care situation would be resolved by the time the kittens moved in, I started playing Borry the sounds of kittens meowing in the hope it would get him used to the idea. I desperately hoped that it would not put his furry nose out of joint. At this point Andrew was now resigned to the fact that

RETURNING FROM A FEW DAYS' SELF-ENFORCED BREAK

I was going slowly insane. (At the time of proof reading this book the two kittens are a year old –– I believe in cat terms that makes them juniors and old Borry died during the Covid-19 lockdown –– they did, however, become the best of buddies).

We had a care agency
They promised it all
I guess we were naïve
They took us for a fool

They said they would deliver
Give care wherever needed
But now Hedge is ill in hospital
That point they've now conceded

They've produced a new policy
That doesn't help at all
In fact it only lets them sit there
For Hedge it is quite cruel

The nurses are just so busy
Rushed off their aching feet
It must be mightily frustrating
Seeing the carer on the seat

Hedge needs continuity
Instead he's getting sad

He feels imprisoned
It makes me feel so bad

But we will champion
We will keep up the pace
We will ping off emails
And chase and chase and chase…

Why oh why oh why does the challenge never end? So with a drippy nose and hoarse voice I was on and off the phone, emailing as fast as my fingers could skim across the keyboard and feeling more and more exhausted. I was half blaming myself for having gone away for a few days and not being on the ward. Words fail me.

I spent the weekend of my return willing Monday to arrive, when I desperately hoped for an update as to what exactly was going to happen.

You think your relative is in safe care
When admitted to a ward
But the act of poor communication
Can mean this being flawed

I now come across as moaning
Forever on the phone

RETURNING FROM A FEW DAYS' SELF-ENFORCED BREAK

Getting crosser by the minute
I feel so damn alone

Why don't they listen?
Why don't they just do?
Instead of making excuses
If only they knew

I am exhausted challenging
Following up on care
My patience is growing less
I'm tearing out my hair

So self-care today
Will be a bag of chips
A moment in my mouth
A lifetime on my hips!

Whilst all this had been going on I decided to start trying to lose weight (as explained in more detail later on in the book). My self-care time eating chips was paying its toll on my waistline. In fact the incentive was that when I am at the hospital it is like being on a diet as I can't afford to keep buying the food and can't quite justify eating in front of Hedge if he is feeling unwell. So the self-care for me was to lose (at the very minimum) a stone in weight. The problem is that I am basically quite lazy and climbing the stairs to the floor that Hedge's ward was on was a complete no no, so I was taking the lift. I don't do exercise, we don't mix, a bit like how oil and water does not mix and at my age my excuse is that I have to start preserving my cartilage not wrecking it through being sporty and running up flights of stairs. It sounds like a plausible justification to me. Allowances can be made for those of a stronger constitution who are not inherently lazy and if you should twist your ankle then at least you might be fortunate enough to have a wheelchair to lean on rather than using crutches.

Seeing things as they are

When we returned home from our break away Andrew and I suddenly saw the light. We both realised that the motorhome no longer had a place in our lives. We were for all intents and purposes kidding ourselves that we would travel the world in it and this particular dream was causing us both more frustration. This decision was made easier due to the fact that whilst away the motorhome's side door refused to open which meant we had to climb in and out from the driver's cab. Furthermore the taps/water pump failed to work so we were unable to use the sink, shower or toilet when away. This combination of factors served to add to our reasons to call it a day. Talk about a tent on wheels.

Winding the clock back, the motorhome had been financed to enable Hedge to get away, but we couldn't even get enough staff to fully cover the short break we had just returned from. So we had to ask ourselves the blatant fact as to how exactly we thought we could manage to take Hedge away without care support. Furthermore what would happen if the taps/water pump continued to be problematic or the side door refused to open? How exactly could Hedge get into the motorhome?

To rub salt into our wounds, Andrew and I also had the daily reminder of our large unused five berth motorhome sat on our driveway, growing moss due to lack of use. So we made the decision to sell the motorhome before we ended up having to reinsure and service it. This way we could start afresh with ideas for small breaks away and maybe just maybe it would help us to de-stress by seeing things as they are, rather than dreaming of a life we could never have.

We both felt a weight had been lifted off our minds due to this decision and apart from the many boxes of clutter that are now being stored under our stairs, from the items we had stowed away in the motorhome, we can begin to move on in our lives. As for Little sis, she is quite happy as it means we will look at staying in hotels instead.

Neither of us can believe the amount of time it took to come to this decision. Maybe one day we may recapture our dreams and purchase a small two berth motorhome to tour Europe in (without children), but for now we have more space on our driveway and boxes of clutter to sort. Self-care comes in many guises and this has been a positive bit of self-care for both of us as we were not looking at the bigger picture, we were only dreaming of something unrealistic and when you dream you get let down.

SEEING THINGS AS THEY ARE

Seeing things as they are
Is something we often forget
But finally the light dawned
And this we won't forget

We've realised and have identified
The motorhome was causing stress
Instead of fun holidays away
Our driveway was a mess

We had to offload everything
For yearly habitation checks
Pay for insurance and tax
We certainly had no regrets

Let someone else now enjoy
Let other families have fun
For us our motorhoming years
Are well and truly done

We can look ahead
Not be stuck in the past
Plan other trips away
A decision made at last!

Toilet humour and self-care

Due to Hedge's condition many hours are spent near or in the toilet. This also means me or Andrew near or in the toilet. Not that we wish to be stalking close by a toilet or accompanying Hedge in the toilet. It does make you wonder quite why so-called accessible toilets fail to understand how privacy is still a pleasant attribute to the user of the facility and privacy is hard to secure when your carer has to assist you on and off the toilet. I dread the Radar key toilets. As many carers and people who need to use the accessible toilets are aware, unless you block the entrance then the toilet door can suddenly swing open due to another person attempting to enter using their Radar key to gain access. I would love to see a pull around screen so that a person can sit and do their deed without having the indecency of going to the toilet in full view of a person who is supporting their needs. I usually just turn my back and take a seat on the wheelchair and pretend I am somewhere else.

It is during my many hours sat on Hedge's wheelchair that I have found the most solace in texting my friend. Both of us regard these quiet moments as valuable as we are able to utilize these enforced downtimes to relish in self-care. Texting each other and ignoring where I am is hugely beneficial to help me while away the time. I have been sat in hospital cubicles, portaloos, small so-called hotel disabled friendly loos that barely allow you to turn a wheelchair around and high street store loos with flickering lighting, not to mention spending hours stood outside non-accessible toilets and having to block the view of Hedge on the toilet whilst I enter to provide assistance if and when required. I have also had to ignore people bashing on the door to speed up proceedings. Having had to endure this indignation on behalf of Hedge, I get the strong desire to swing the door open violently as I walk out backwards pulling the wheelchair. I then take pleasure in swinging the wheelchair round with the help of Hedge, whilst I attempt to disguise the smirk on my face, politely apologising for taking our time.

I did once try to add up the amount of time assisting in this way and it equated to over a year of my life (so far). I feel frustrated at wasting time spent in this way, but what about poor Hedge for whom numerous health professionals over the years have said he spends too much time on the toilet and even equated sitting on the toilet to being behavioural! Fortunately now in adult services the health professionals are more understanding and compassionate, appreciating that due to Hedge's complex gastric problems this simple activity of daily living can be a prolonged and exhausting experience for Hedge. The Gastroenterology Team are amazing in adult services and see Hedge for who he is rather than fobbing him off that there is nothing wrong. Hedge is now on medication to help his gastric system to work better and we no longer have to challenge for help in this way. It is sad that it took 18 years for Hedge to be properly managed in this way, but this has in some way been a success in his transition to adult services.

Grab those moments
When you don't expect
Take each opportunity
No one will detect

Whether it be in a toilet
Or hovering just outside
Have downtime to treasure
And lots more beside

Don't think of the place
Just think of the time
Text a good friend
It isn't a crime

Catch up on a chat
Google away
Send an emoji
Pass the time of day

Once the task is done
Carry on as before
Your catch ups well done
Toileting no longer a chore!

Fabrications and little lies

I can assure the reader that all fabrications and white lies are not mine. They appear from nowhere and grow bigger like tumbleweed and get more and more unbelievably incredulous each time someone recalls, writes or mentions them. I grow tired of the constant battles (or challenges as Andrew likes to call them) in order for Hedge to be provided with a service and not be discriminated against due to his rare condition not being acknowledged by many who could make his life easier by recognising that Hedge is who he is rather than putting up a new Berlin Wall each time he is referred their way.

I do however find that self-care comes in many guises and I love the satisfaction of typing up a letter in counter defence of some obscure report that is full of ambiguous information. It is so gratifying getting things down in writing and either posting a reply or pinging off an email that you know will cause aggro due to the information you have supplied being correct. A Solicitor of ours once wrote letters by email that would arrive at 3pm on a Friday afternoon to create as much impact as possible to the person receiving it. The Solicitor's letters were particularly heart-warming when you knew that it would cause grief as she had requested responses tied to a legal timeframe. Alas, I can't do that, but I can bash out a letter in reply to a load of nonsense very quickly. Vexingly I am also aware that the big-guns of organisations will stick together like glue in order to protect each other, regardless of whether they are incorrect. The small fry like me are easily brushed aside as many won't even bother to challenge, many can't and some people haven't the ability to know how to complain or get justice for their loved ones.

>
> Fabrications and little lies
> Where do I begin?
> I was always taught to be honest
> As being disingenuous is a sin
>
> Yet I see the letters written
> As I read the words within
> Where is the information from?
> It's not a game to win
>
> I read each and every page
> Growing red in disbelief
> I feel quite nauseated
> All I see is grief
>
> I know I cannot rest
> I cannot let this go
> How can the powers that be
> Find time to sink so low?

I need to reply
I need to set things straight
I have plenty of evidence
I need to shut that gate

So carefully I compose
A letter back in return
Evidencing each wrong statement
Showing they've lots to learn

Transition is a joke
For Hedge it's gone so wrong
Let's hope I can make things better
And it doesn't take too long

So yet again I post off
A letter to explain
That the facts they are quoting
Are simply wrong again!

Mother's Day with the Brownies

I am not a religious person, I have faith in karma and whilst I used to be a choir girl, I now attend Church to support Little sis when she attends services for Brownies. It was on one such occasion that I had no care cover for Hedge once again, so told him that he would have to attend Church with me. Now Hedge either does or doesn't do the whole Church thing depending on his mood, but on this occasion he happily agreed to attend as it was for Mother's Day and he wished to see Little sis in her Brownie uniform.

We go to sit down and instantly realise that unless Hedge sits in his wheelchair stuck out in the aisle, then I will have to transfer him to the Church pew. Therefore I manage to get Hedge to sit beside me and we are instantly made to feel unwelcome by the lady sat in front who is bemoaning the fact and loudly muttering why so many people have bothered to turn up today, when they usually don't bother. I start talking rather loudly about anything to drown out the crabby old lady's voice. The lady is evidently not going to shut up anytime soon and what with Hedge asking me a hundred and one questions I feel like my hour in Church is going to be a very long hour indeed. It is with pleasure that I say I need not have worried, as I got the best self-care in the world and when I least expected it! It is safe to say that I have not laughed so much in a very long time and quite how I managed to stifle my laughter is beyond me.

It all started during the hymns. Hedge loves singing. Hedge also wholeheartedly loves getting into singing, with the whole arm movements and extra swirly bits at the end of lines. It should have been simple, a quick hymn or two, listen to the sermon and then across the road over to the Church hall for refreshments. Only Hedge had other ideas with his extra loud, extra out of tune rendition of 'Morning has Broken'. Oh my goodness Hedge totally got into it and his voice was soon very much louder than the annoying lady in front of us and she turned around showing such a look of distaste that I instantly choked and from then on sniggered and sniggered and chuckled my way through the rest of the hymn. Hedge was in his element and visibly very much enjoying it. Hedge's finale was the extra-long 'yeah' he sung out of tune at the end!

My poor nose was running and tears were streaming down my face as an annoyed Little sis handed over the posy of flowers that the Brownies were giving out! The more I tried not to laugh the more I set myself off and the thought of the irate lady in front of me just made it worse. I then had my last laugh when at the end of the Church Service I went to get the wheelchair and stopped the annoying irate lady from leaving her pew as

I purposely took extra-long getting Hedge settled into it. I felt like a naughty school child and free from the worries of the world as I sauntered out of Church that day!

>
> Grab it where you can
> A tiny laugh or two
> Who cares where you are
> Be it at home or in a pew
>
> Let the sniggers out
> Wipe your tears away
> Be grateful for your laughter
> As it brightens up your day!

Decluttering for self-care

Who would have ever thought it, I succumbed to purchasing some wonder powder to get my whites extra white. The local supermarket was selling it half price so I thought I would give it a go. However, I first needed to dig out suitable items to be trialled whilst using it. So I had a fab plan of decluttering my chest of drawers. I discovered a suspender belt from 1990 that refused to go around my thigh. Strangely enough in 1990 I don't recall thinking I was particularly slim, but apparently I must have been because however much I tried to stretch the damn thing, it refused to grow any bigger and get anywhere near my stomach. So much for my hope of feeling better on decluttering. As for the suspender belt it headed straight for the bin. Next I found two dingy white slightly too small bras and an old maternity one. Goodness knows why I was keeping these, but I decided they could become part of my experiment and I could dunk them in the wonder stuff and pull them out glowing white. I therefore finished chucking out 26 pairs of way too small knickers, goodness knows how many pairs of tights that had undoubtedly seen their best days and half a dozen pairs of socks. Feeling chuffed with the way the drawers were now closing (without me having to ram them in place); I trotted off downstairs to mix up the potion that would give me glowing white undergarments!

So here goes, I dip in the bra, but decide to keep one half in and one half out to get the full magical effect of the whiteness (as shown in the adverts). Only nothing happens. I therefore move on to the next white item I have plundered from the laundry basket and end up reaching for my 99 pence magnifying glasses to see if I can spot a difference. Nope, what's in the sink still looks grubby. I then add more of the wonder powder and leave it for half an hour whilst I get myself a coffee. I go back to the sink, lift up the now thoroughly soaked items of clothing and still no difference. So I grab the lot and quickly shove it all in the washing machine. I add more of the wonder powder and stick the whole lot on a wash.

Fast forward one and a half hours and I go to the washing machine that is bleeping like crazy to tell me the cycle has ended and, full of anticipation, open the door and remove the clothing. The results were woefully less impressive than I had thought and the wire of the bra is now stuck in the drum of the machine. By the time I get off the kitchen floor after prising the wire out of the drum I feel like a little old lady as I can barely stand. Irksomely I am now holding one wonky bra, a wire from the bra and the whole lot still looked grubby. Was it a waste of a day? Not entirely, as I succeeded in clearing out my chest of drawers and had fun experimenting with the so called whiter than white powder. Next time I shall just walk on by and not bother purchasing any bargains to trial. I could have used bleach at a fraction of the price and probably have received better results. Now just maybe I should find my bleach and give it another go…

I am a sucker for a bargain
I like to try things new
But rarely do I get it right
The claims are never true

I go out shopping for one thing
And come back laden down
My new gadgets rarely work
Andrew looks and wears a frown

It is a five minute wonder
It really is a crime
I get roped in with an offer
Each and every time

So next time you are shopping
And see a bargain on the shelf
Don't bother there's no point
You'll just wind up yourself

Your shopping will be cheaper
If you listen to my mistake
Your self-care more fulfilling
If you just buy cake!

The tragic case of mistaken communication

It is extremely sad to say that due to a situation that occurred on the ward where Hedge was an inpatient, it resulted in a safeguarding alert being raised. The whole circumstance could have been very much avoided if Hedge's carers from the agency had been supporting instead of refusing to provide the care they were commissioned to provide. However, due to huge gaps in the provision from the commissioned care agency, a foreign agency worker employed by the hospital kindly offered to give Hedge a shower. It is deeply regretful that due to a complete breakdown of understanding on Hedge's part and the health care assistant speaking English as a second language that they both misunderstood what was being said and the whole conversation left Hedge deeply distressed. I tried for many hours to reassure Hedge that it was probably due to his understanding and communication issues, but Hedge was inconsolable, so I reluctantly asked for us to speak to the Ward Sister. I thought that was the end of it until the Safeguarding Nurse for the hospital asked to speak to Hedge together with the Ward Manager. I was mortified as being a nurse myself I knew that the poor agency worker would have also been questioned and was probably feeling dreadful further to this occurring. The only point the investigation highlighted was the need for Hedge to have his own carers support him, so that incidents like this would be mitigated. Only, due to the lack of carers available from the care agency this would be unlikely to happen. This meant that during times when I should have been enjoying self-care I was now stuck in the hospital attempting to ensure that Hedge's voice was being heard, so that the staff could start to thoroughly understand him. The frustration on my part was growing bigger as I could see how important it was that Hedge was able to be validated as having a learning disability but due to the ridiculous scenario with the Learning Disability Team declining him, it was undeniably leaving Hedge extremely vulnerable. Therefore the team who were happily delivering care for patients with learning disabilities were in fact discriminating against Hedge as he was being left far more exposed and vulnerable than any other patient who had a learning disability would ever be, or indeed anyone else for that matter. This is something I still can't get my head around.

Taking a positive spin on the situation, it did mean that we were now talking to the person in charge rather than those who did not have the authority to make a decision and this in itself was comforting.

Hence my self-care whilst sat beside Hedge was hoping that Hedge would nod off to sleep for 30 minutes so that I could read a book and enjoy drinking the coffee that the lady from

THE TRAGIC CASE OF MISTAKEN COMMUNICATION

the Hotel Services kindly gave me when the trolley came round. I am adept at grabbing every opportunity and these quick five minutes of 'me time' supported me to get through some tough days on the ward.

Communication is a must
Getting it wrong will never do
But if carers don't understand
They'll end up in a stew

The carer communicates one thing
Hedge will receive it wrong
They'll both go around the houses
Wondering why it takes so long

The answers are given
Both think they've got it right
But actually both are incorrect
Almost there but somehow not quite

In the end Hedge gets distressed
The carer can't work out why
They both get in a pickle
And I just want to cry

I see how Hedge communicates
His processing speed too slow

'THE UNOFFICIAL SELF-CARE GUIDE FOR CARERS'

His short-term memory is diabolical
Meaning communication doesn't flow

I get the jargon and the slang
I see where it goes wrong
But when you communicate with Hedge
Simple questions go on and on

You can go around in circles
It wears you down in time
With the main problem being
Communication as the crime

Don't just assume or ignore
Think about what is said
That way you'll both stay on track
And you won't end up seeing red

Rising early to attempt self-care

Having been squashed overnight by Borry who had once again decided to lie across my feet, I wake up feeling squashed and with a painful leg. It is plainly obvious that the giant furball that feels as heavy as a sack of potatoes wishes me to get up as he is now purring loudly in my ear and looking like he is going to swipe everything off my bedside cabinet. I am not the type of person who only has an alarm clock and placemat for a glass of water, I have a bedside cabinet that resembles a jumble sale containing everything I might need if there was nuclear warfare declared overnight. Whilst I digress, I do wonder how many people's homes genuinely look like the ones shown on TV adverts as however much I tidy up it still looks messy. So back to what I was meant to be writing about, I gingerly get up –– thanks, cat for making my feet feel heavy and tired. I have a shower which takes an age to come on due to poor water pressure and hear the cat meowing and scratching the bathroom door. I speed along my so-called relaxing shower, aware that my rather annoying feline friend is about to wake Andrew and Little sis. Therefore, still dripping wet I grab a towel to wrap around me and call the cat into the bathroom and instantly regret this decision as he decides to circle my legs and rub himself against me. Great, so I am now covered in cat fur and the black jeggings I have in mind will be covered when I try to pull them over my feet. I valiantly fend off the cat that is by now becoming an annoyance and put back on my PJ bottoms to save any issues with cat fur. I so wish cats didn't moult.

I sneak downstairs and look up at the church clock which is clearly visible from my kitchen window and see that it is still only 06:30 hours. I make myself a coffee, water the garden (it was looking rather dry), put a load of washing on, put a new ironing board cover on the ironing board (how come if it goes one way round it is too big and the other it is too small). This simple task takes me in excess of 20 minutes and I am cursing by the time it is almost achieved, having found some old nappy pins to get it to semi fit. I then check my emails and to my relief see that I don't need to collect the kittens until next weekend. It gives me a reprieve of another weekend where I don't have to be monitoring the activities of the kittens and my large furry friend that I already have. Then I just sit and chill. I tried to put the TV on but the remote is refusing to play ball, so I sit and feel guilty to the point that after only about a minute I get up and decide to do some cleaning.

Ok, so my attempt at rising early for self-care has rather flummoxed me. I truly can't relax. I need to be doing something, otherwise I am stressing about the situation with Hedge being in hospital again. My mind simply cannot switch off. I suppose

RISING EARLY TO ATTEMPT SELF-CARE

that is why I find gardening so therapeutic as I can hack away to my heart's delight, keep busy and achieve something tangible. I find housework boring (I am sure I am not alone in disliking housework) and as for sorting the post, where does it all come from and why do I need so much? There is a permanent pile on my kitchen cabinet waiting for me to go through.

A new attempt at self-care
Rising early to be alone
No calls for help with homework
No hard sales on the phone

Instead the cat's demanding
There's washing-up in the sink
There's laundry for the machine
I grab a quick coffee to drink

The church clock tells me
It's only half past six
If only I knew how to relax
Whilst I hoof down my Weetabix

There's a pile of post waiting
I need to sort and bin
I feel as guilty as anything
I really cannot win

'THE UNOFFICIAL SELF-CARE GUIDE FOR CARERS'

Relaxing's not for me
I get more stressed instead
I might have well gone back to sleep
Or read a book in bed!

Starting a new course

After many years getting nowhere with regards to Hedge's support, I have been perfectly aware that I cannot afford for Little sis to suffer any ill-gotten consequences due to the lack of Hedge's support. Little sis is ferociously bright, but this brings a weight upon her shoulders and we know that she struggles with friendships, probably due to her having a 'wise head on young shoulders' and growing up quickly due to also caring for Hedge. I attempted to get school involved many years ago, but we found a lot of the support was very piecemeal. So due to the fear of us hitting the teen years head on without any ideas on how to manage, I enrolled on a 'Therapeutic Parenting' course. I was rather under the impression that this would instantly solve all problems, which it didn't. However, it did allow me a 45-minute drive to the venue and the chance to sit and listen to the radio whilst driving there and back. The sitting and listening during the course was more intense than I had initially thought and I sat there going through shopping lists in my head and having to snap myself back to what the leader of the course was talking about. I also struggled hearing all about everyone else's problems. I very much doubted I would make a close friendship with any of the other course attendees as suggested on day one, as I have limited time to see Andrew, let alone strum up a meaningful relationship with someone else who also has a truck load of problems. I knew I had enough on my plate already. I very much hoped that maybe my initial enthusiasm for attending the course might have got reignited, so I waited patiently for a change to occur. It is now obvious to me that having grown rhino skin over the years, my patience for life continues to decrease. I presume I am now bordering on, if not already, in the grumpy old woman stage in life.

During session number one we had to introduce ourselves as though we were the child we had come to learn how to parent therapeutically. I did tell Little sis afterwards how I introduced the family through her eyes and it was quite insightful seeing her reaction. She said I got most of it right, but told me that she would never have said what I did for a job as it was not 'significant'! Keeping an open mind about looking through a child's eyes I tried doing this through Hedge's eyes and oh my goodness it made me sit back and take stock of how testing life is for Hedge. It is all very fine me breezing up to the hospital, bringing clean clothes and a smiling face, but for Hedge he is stuck there day in day out, bored and alone. No wonder he is forever phoning me asking me for my advice. Hedge is like a 20 year old man in a ten year old's body and the fact that the powers that be are denying him the support he so desperately needs continues to destroy my hope in humanity.

STARTING A NEW COURSE

I tried therapeutic parenting
To try to help me cope
I thought it would be simple
Like selling old rope

But instead my easy course
Made me sit up and think
It questioned all my parenting
And made my stomach sink

It made me see
How all those years ago
I should have sought more help
To enable Hedge to flourish and grow

But all those years ago
When I asked and sought support
All I ever got
Was another damn report

So now my parenting skills
Will be well and truly honed (I hope)
To provide Little sis with help
My parenting ability more toned

I remember something similar
So many moons ago

But it was far less course content
And when you reap you sow

I clearly forgot a lot I learnt
So here's to renewing knowledge
I can enthusiastically utilise my skills
To help Little sis and Hedge!

It was therefore no surprise that I did not form any meaningful relationship with any of the other parents attending the course. I do, however, now look at situations from either Little Sis's or Hedge's eyes before I go in all cross and quite often it helps me alter the way I approach them. I really like role play and also use this to show how they are being when they are driving me up the wall and it is surprising how it calms the situation. Yes, they do think I am mad, but I would far rather act like a mad person for a five minute break then let them carry on making me feel insane for hours.

The tale of two kittens (who are utterly adorable)

Yet another of my crazy moments of madness was in agreeing to Hedge having two kittens, and this became a reality. I mentioned it earlier in the book (just dropped it in there to see if anyone was paying attention to detail in what I have been writing). I had been suckered in and have now paid the price for my love of cats. I was therefore left having visions of splitting up Borry from them and also dreams of them snuggling all together on the bed. I was apprehensive and nervous of this new venture, especially as Hedge was in hospital with no light at the end of the tunnel for him to come home anytime soon. The agency he had, had also just been served 28 days' notice and the new agency still had to recruit to post.

In the meantime, I had kittens arriving. Their breed is known to be hypoallergenic so there will be no excuse for future carers to say that they are allergic to cats. I had once again fallen for Hedge's needing for a pet hook, line and sinker. Mercifully I am a huge cat lover so when he went on and on and on for kittens, I knew I would be unable to resist. In all fairness we did seek out rescue cats first, but the only one a local shelter felt was suitable for Hedge was a one eyed, shy skinny cat that had just flown in from Dubai. I did feel sorry for it, but it hardly had the cute factor Hedge was after and he was rather scared of touching it due to the way the cat looked at him. It rather reminded me of the 'That's Life' episode of the stuffed cat (for anyone who remembers TV from the 1980s). Frustratingly Andrew is a dog person and was not that overenthusiastic about the fact that the kittens were coming to live at our house until Hedge returned home. Andrew also constantly kindly reminded me that poor old Borry would have his nose put out of joint when they arrived.

I could see the negative and the positives in the whole situation. The negative being I would be the one having to sort their litter trays and be the person who prevents world war three from occurring when they didn't get on with my cat. The positive was that they will be bigger when Hedge returned home so that he will not accidently squeeze them too tightly, due to his poor hand-eye co-ordination. The hospital had also agreed that I could take them in to visit Hedge if they are on a leash. I imagined getting a few odd stares but apparently this breed of cat is more like a dog and described as a dog in cats' fur. So fingers crossed I hoped that all would go to plan.

In the meantime, Hedge had been busy purchasing items online for the kittens and I kept getting rather large deliveries. Little sis and myself spent a Sunday afternoon putting together the biggest cat tree in the world of cat trees. When I was a child I don't think scratching posts had even been invented and my cat used to spend his life scratching a post in my parents' hallway and my mother would be forever re-wallpapering it so my father would not find out. My mother ended up deciding to paint the post instead, which put an end to the scratching of the wallpaper. As for the cat tree Hedge purchased, it was huge and I had to stand on a chair to get the last bit in place. Andrew came home and was not at all impressed about the newest item in our kitchen-diner and asked "…and what is that?" I politely replied, "A cat tree." As good fortune had it, Borry quickly got used to the added bits in the house and I hoped that just adding in two kittens would not be too much of a shock as he had already seen the new extra-large hooded litter tray, new bed, cat toys, feeding bowls etc.

One night before they arrived and after Little sis was in bed, I decided to put together the cat circuit toy that was Hedge's latest purchase. I put the box on my kitchen table and sat down with a lovely hot cup of coffee. I anticipated getting a real sense of satisfaction and some well-deserved self-care time as I enjoy putting things together. Only, the task was more difficult than I had thought. Firstly, I couldn't read the instructions and had to go on a hunt for a pair of my reading glasses. I have four pairs in total and my coffee was cold by the time I found them. The instructions meticulously explained that you can make the circuit up in many different combinations to help keep cats entertained and to provide enrichment. Great, so it should be relatively simple; however, try as I might each time I clipped the pieces in place, it was pretty obvious that it was never going to make a circuit. By now I was becoming frustrated and the thought of feeling good about having completed a task was far from my mind. Muttering furiously to myself about what a ridiculous cat toy Hedge had bought, I wrenched the whole thing apart and put it back in the box. I then had a lightbulb moment and looked on the box at the picture and saw that I was one piece missing. Exasperatingly this was the reason for me fiddling around for an hour trying to make sense of the instructions and getting nowhere fast. As I pushed back on the chair to go and hunt for the receipt, my foot hit a piece that I had dropped whilst tipping the pieces out on the table. I could have screamed. So, I tipped out the other pieces and made the circuit for a final time. I then proceeded to try to show my ginger furry friend what to do with the circuit toy and was annoyed when he promptly turned around and walked off!

The funniest bit that made me laugh out loud was the next morning when Little sis was late at the breakfast table. I went to go and get her only to hear her playing with the cat circuit toy, so called upstairs in a surprised voice "Oh my goodness I didn't realise the kittens had arrived overnight!" The reply came back "They are not here, Mum, I am practising." Practising, what exactly is Little sis practising for? Unless of course she is going to spend hours showing the kittens what to do. I imagine they will turn their noses up and walk off too. Maybe I should have kept the box and taken it back to the pet shop after all.

THE TALE OF TWO KITTENS (WHO ARE UTTERLY ADORABLE)

Hedge has done it again
I've been suckered right in
My ability to say no
Meant only Hedge could win

At first it was one kitten
Then one became two
He said they'll keep each other company
And that is very true

Only I didn't expect
Hedge not to be at home
Meaning I'd have them all the time
So in my house they'll roam

My poor old ginger tomcat
Will probably be upset
I truly hope the kittens behave
And that I don't regret

Andrew suggested a dog
Can you really imagine me?
Trying to train man's best friend
Training pads full of poo and wee

I have convinced myself
Without sight of a moan or shout

> The kittens were meant to be
> Somehow it will all work out!

Self-care is a curious thing, but I truly anticipated that having two kittens for a while would help me relax when I was cuddling them. However, I was slightly intrepid at the thought of them scratching our new leather sofa, which now sported a big fabric protector on it. Andrew kept reminding me about the fact we had saved up for a leather sofa, only we couldn't see it anymore due to the newly purchased fabric covers. Begrudgingly I might just agree with him on that one, but I strongly sensed it was for the best as if and when the kittens scratched the leather sofa Andrew would be none the wiser as he would have got used to the fabric protectors!

Self-care and pets is something I simply cannot provide my pennyworth on. Dog lovers, cat lovers, bearded dragon lovers, we all get hoodwinked and end up taking more on than we would like to admit. I have been duped like all of us are who own a family pet.

Eating healthily (finally) to lose weight

I had long ago decided that having seen so much death in my work as a Community Nurse, that I would eat what I want, when I want without feeling guilty. However, a time came when I saw myself as I was. My realisation moment came when I had squeezed myself into a pair of lovely summer blue jeans that required a belt. I took the belt out of my wardrobe and was shocked to find that I could not even do up the last hole in the belt. I had a huge wobbly muffin top escaping over the top of my jeans. I struggled to do the belt up feeling quite crippled, but decided to put a baggy jumper over the top. Oh dear, I had regrettably not checked the mirror before I left home, as when I arrived at the hospital and got in the empty lift the mirror opposite me showed an aging woman who had completely lost the plot regarding her weight and had been completely overindulging.

This revelation was the shock I needed to kickstart my healthy eating plan. Much to my annoyance and competitive streak, Andrew had experienced the same with his belt and therefore we both hit the healthy eating plan at the same time. Fortunately,

I have a savoury tooth, so my cravings for sugary cakes and biscuits are minimal. Unfortunately for Andrew, he often works away and eats out a lot. However, this had given me the boost I needed as I could find no better way in promoting my own self-care than beating Andrew in the weight stakes. In three weeks I had lost 13 pounds in weight and was feeling much healthier as a consequence. The weight came off easily to begin with, but I soon found I was having to do the one legged stand on the scales to ensure they showed the number I wanted them to show. I weighed my handbag and it weighed six pounds and there was no greater feeling than seeing how I had lost twice this amount. I aimed to be fab by fifty and only had six weeks to go. I was a woman with a mission and genuinely felt fab already as I could now get my belt done up on the third hole along. Sadly, I can only do it up to hole number two now, but the good food I have eaten putting the weight back on has been worth it!

I also allowed myself some not so healthy treats and had fish and chips when I wanted and even the odd cream tea and still the weight came off! I was surprised to find the cream tea too sweet so decided to give any future ones a miss, but I never gave up on indulging in my love for chips. Little sis was also loving the competition between her mum and dad and cheekily asked who had won. Fortunately for us, Little sis loves her fruit and vegetables, so we were not subjected to watching her eat tasty treats whilst having to ignore what she was munching on.

You have to be happy living in the skin you are in, but when something about the skin you are in is making you unhappy then change it. Some women love to colour their hair, it makes them feel good. For me colouring my hair became a monthly Sunday morning ritual that took up far too much time and I actually became happier when I embraced the grey. Some people I know thought I had it coloured that way, but I can assure everyone it is completely natural. I have more time, more money in my purse and now relish the grey. I strongly consider that far too many people live their lives worried about how others perceive them, but actually who gives a fig about your hair colour. Embrace the colour you love, but do not let it take over your life like I had. I distinctly remember how stressed I would get if I saw the pesky grey parting line starting to appear. Now I have one less stress and no wasted Sundays.

The fact that Andrew was beginning to slip on the weight front was like music to my ears. Having been away so much for work meant that he was eating out too much and too many meals out meant the pounds were going back on. I, on the other hand, had lost a whopping 24 pounds and when I saw my reflection in the mirrored hospital lift on the way to Hedge's ward, I only saw a bit of a bulge, where I had previously seen a completely sagging double tyre. As the lift was empty apart from Little sis and myself I did a daft dance in front of the mirror much to Little sis's embarrassment. It was just such a great 'self-care' feeling that I almost looked forward to getting back into the lift again to smile at my newly acquired slimmer me.

'THE UNOFFICIAL SELF-CARE GUIDE FOR CARERS'

Dieting and fads, I've done it all
From fasting and calorie counting
Slimming teas and magic pills
However, the pounds kept mounting

Then one day I saw a reflection of me
A double tyre for a middle and chin
Quite bloated and clothes not looking good
Clearly my chips had been more than just a sin

My muffin top spilling over my jeans
Looking frumpy, tired and just a tad old
Left me staring at a much older version of me
I guess Andrew never said as he wasn't that bold

So it was left down to me to see for myself
That I needed to get a grip and do some self-care
Taking care of myself and not overindulging
Looking healthier and slimmer with greying hair

I have a treat and chips just once a week
Have cut back on the savouries and wine
And got used to feeling a little less full
In order to take back control of that flab of mine!

Passing the hot potato

This is a saying that I now speak about a lot. I speak about it to my friends, who also feel the same and to other care workers and professionals that Andrew and I meet at the many meetings we attend on Hedge's behalf. It is almost as though professionals can't wait to assess Hedge, produce a report (often citing incorrect facts) and then wipe their hands clean, grateful that they can fob Hedge off for another day. More recently, Hedge has swiftly moved from having significant mental health needs requiring therapy, to not having any needs other than having an 'emerging personality disorder' and now it has become a 'well-known borderline personality disorder'. Strange as it may seem, Andrew, Hedge and I have not heard that the emerging personality disorder had now become a well-known borderline personality disorder. Furthermore, the meeting between the outgoing Child Psychiatrist (who advised Hedge had very different needs) and the Adult Psychiatrist (who totally disagreed) still needs to happen in order to discuss who is right and who is wrong. Their contradicting viewpoints are so far apart that we were half expecting to be told that they had both spoken about a different person. It would certainly not be the first time this has happened as when Hedge was a child under Great Ormond Street, a Consultant was once 20 minutes into his appointment before he and we realised he was speaking about the wrong child. Calling Hedge by the wrong name was a bit of a big clue into this error. However, on this occasion the Psychiatrists are speaking about the same person and Andrew and myself are wondering whether this is due to the adult mental health service not having the capacity to take Hedge on and is more about saving money than being needs-led. However, Andrew and I have now been assured that a meeting between all parties will be convened so they can get to the bottom of the very differing opinions. It just makes me wonder how many other people have been wrongly told they don't have any mental health needs when they clearly do.

So back to passing the hot potato, it appeared that the Urology team who dealt with Hedge's urinary problems also attempted to pass the hot potato when they failed to attend to an urgent request by the medical team to see Hedge on the ward for a blocked catheter. By which time Hedge had to have a significant amount of pain relief and anti-sickness. Fortunately for me I had pre-empted the significant delay by the Urology team and already raised a formal complaint highlighting the risks of a urine infection alongside many other issues that would happen as a result of not attending to the blocked catheter in a timely manner. It perplexed me that in the community a nurse could replace the type of catheter Hedge had, but in the hospital I had been told that only a doctor could. This was even more frustrating for me as I have replaced hundreds of these as a nurse, yet had to watch Hedge suffer so much because no-one in the hospital could do this in a timely manner. Then just as I had foreseen, Hedge ended up with a urine infection requiring intravenous antibiotics.

To say my blood was boiling is an understatement. In the interim I pinged off many emails, finding this a cathartic way of getting my frustrations out and also a tiny bit of self-care as it forced me to sit down for five minutes with a cup of coffee whilst I typed away leaving a very clear audit trail.

In all honesty I don't know what the answer is regarding Hedge's care in hospital as unless Hedge has one-to-one support to advocate his needs constantly, then his needs are not effectively met. Hedge's inability to express himself properly due to not listening effectively in the first place makes things very complex for anyone trying to care for him. Having recently watched another shocking report about abuse in the care system, I dread being no longer around to advocate when Hedge is desperate for a listening ear that will result in the listening ear not being too intimidated to stand up for his rights. Abuse takes many guises and due to staffing shortages care staff can understandably struggle to deliver safe, consistent care. Subtle lapses in Hedge's care, create a domino effect of other issues cropping up. These issues compound in a chain reaction of other events amounting to Hedge needing more care which the staff are then up against trying to provide and so the snowball effect continues. It is then a challenge to untangle the resultant problems and backward chain to what really occurred.

Therefore, as a carer, the question was, did I go into hospital when I could or step back to demonstrate how demanding Hedge's care needs continue to be? That is a tricky question as when I go in I am quickly frustrated by Hedge's thousands of demands and constant wish to bicker, and I go home drained and grumpy when caring for Little sis. So through practising tough love I only visited for a few hours at a time. I could have visited more but failed to see why I should deliver all the care and don't get as much as a biscuit in return. I then have to watch as the food from the mealtime trolley is thrown away because the catering staff are not allowed to give any unused food to a carer. All the while I am hungry and thirsty and either pay the highly overinflated cost of food in the hospital or stay hungry and thirsty. Not quite what I need to assist with my self-care. Many may say take something with you, but when I am already spinning plates in the air the last thing I need is to then have to get up even earlier in the morning to make myself sandwiches, whilst endeavouring to shimmy Little sis along to make sure she gets to school on time.

> Pass the hot potato
> Is a game I'd love to play
> My son's needs are too complex
> So park him for the day
>
> I'll fob off and write a letter
> I'll use jargon to confuse

PASSING THE HOT POTATO

I'll let someone else stress
And his care I'll just refuse

I'll email late on Friday
Just before I go away
That will save a bit of time
And waste another day

I'll only have the young adult
Who looks easy to care for
That young person's too demanding
So I'll simply close the door

Gosh wouldn't life be fab
If I could play the game
I'd pass Hedge like a hot potato
And never speak his name

But oddly enough I'm Mum
I can't play that silly game
I've got to keep on going
As I can't live with that shame

However, I will ping off emails
Ask questions about his care
Happily sit in and advocate at meetings
And raise concerns and share

Seeing into the future

It appears that it is not only myself that wishes to look deep into the future, but Hedge also has this same desire. I used to avidly read my stars in the women's magazines I used to buy when I was younger and did try out seeing a clairvoyant and even a medium. I might have been sceptical about the medium before I saw her, but I held very different views on leaving. Looking back I can see that she was very right about many things in my life, other than my children. The medium did say I would become a nurse and would end up with a man who was living miles away. I never breathed a word to the medium about either my boyfriend at the time who was Andrew, who was living over 200 miles away or the fact that I had always wanted to be a nurse.

The recently purchased fortune telling ball remains in use and kindly provides me with the answers I want after I repeatedly shake it to ensure I get the final answer I am after. This is all a bit of fun, but it strengthened Hedge's resolve to see another Clairvoyant, having already seen one a few months ago. I have to say the previous one's predictions were not great as she told Hedge that his health would improve this year and be much better. Hedge has now been researching and wants to go along to one that is more highly recommended. However what Hedge is truly seeking is the knowledge that he is going to be ok and have a partner for life. I am unclear whether this can ever be answered for him.

It saddens me that society naturally appears to assume (correct me if I am wrong) that someone like Hedge will end up partnered with another person who has a disability. Hedge has been referred to only social groups for people with disabilities. Maybe just maybe Hedge might like to attend something non-disabled. Is it too hard to accept that he won't end up partnering someone not in a wheelchair? OK so I get it that sporting events need to be suited to the ability of the person, but what about other clubs? Over and over again, people with disabilities get overlooked. I once tried to book a seat to see a famous London Theatre show that had come to our local theatre and was devastated when I was told that the seats we would normally book were no longer available due to the cast needing them. Therefore we missed the show as these were the seats normally allocated for wheelchair users.

The partner for life and adult social groups were not even considered when Hedge was a child. Why would I even think about these issues? Life was so much less complicated. Society pretends to care, but does it really? Services are so tightly ringfenced that it leaves people like Hedge even more vulnerable than the people who have a protected need such as a learning disability. Time and time again Hedge's needs are failed and he suffers due to those around him not understanding his vulnerabilities. Making reasonable adjustments is a legal requirement for someone with a learning disability, yet there are no reasonable adjustments made for Hedge. Actually, it gives rise to the question as to whether services should ensure that the same high quality of care and adjustments should be made for everyone, not just for a select group in society. This is especially important when the criteria for being validated as having a learning disability is so inconsistent and not everyone has an IQ test. Some people are automatically accepted due to their disability or chromosome abnormality, whereas others are not. It's like saying if you are 5 ft. tall then you qualify for a stool to stand on to help you see over heads of the football fans at the football match, but if you are 5 ft. and ¼ inch you don't qualify for a stool to stand on so you do not see any of the match. How exactly would that be seen as an equitable service? Services can be so ringfenced that they become blinkered to the actual needs of society, which in my opinion just serves to discriminate and make those who are a tiny bit outside the criteria worse off then those who meet the criteria.

Hence the need for a clairvoyant to foretell the future and save Hedge the hassle of second guessing all the time. I actually quite like the idea of going along too as maybe they could let me know whether or not I will ever get a day when I am not constantly worried about Hedge. Now that would be a great bit of self-care. I could sit and chill out whilst being told all the positive things in my life that are about to happen, as Clairvoyants tend not to tell you anything bad. It could be a great pick-me-up and I could go home ignoring the real stuff going on. Or maybe not!

I wish I could foretell
What future was in store?
All positive I hope
Else my chin would hit the floor

I'd like to see great things
Achievements far and wide
Not all the stress and worry
A thorn stabbing in my side

I could be told great news
Hedge will have a great life
Not sitting on his own
No more sadness or strife

That crystal ball will see
Lots of self-care and fun
Not the constant snacking
Because I'm always on the run

It might cost me a bit
When I hand over the money
I am happy to pay anything
If they predict a life of milk and honey

But regretfully I know
Deep down in my soul
That even a clairvoyant
Will struggle predicting my role

I'd sit there handing over money
Making shopping lists in my head
Wishing I'd had a bag of chips
And paid for something else instead!

Juggling my life away

Like many carers I spend my day juggling the trials of each day and attempting to make some kind of order in my mind. My work keeps me sane and allows me valuable time-out from the constant daily demands of being a carer. I really don't know how I would cope if I did not have something else to focus my mind on. This serves to add to my dose of self-care that is so important for enabling me to keep going.

I was at the hospital visiting Hedge on one occasion and ended up being with him for the best part of the day due to him being so out of sorts again. I took ten minutes to chat to the lady visiting her husband in the bed opposite and she told me how she used to be a carer in a residential home before she retired. This charming lady spoke a lot of sense and reminded me of the value of taking time to care for myself. She had spent most of her working years dedicated to care of the elderly, yet dreaded becoming old herself due to the perceived lack of time available by the younger generation to actually care. We stood there like a couple of book ends sharing our frustrations about care today and whilst we stood there we realised that most of the patients had no sheets on their beds. Unfortunately the health care worker had stripped all the beds and then realised that no linen had been sent up to the ward. We also realised that none of the patients in the bay had received a mid-morning drink. We could have picked fault with so much of the care that day, but had to remind ourselves that the ward was chaotic and terribly understaffed and a lot of the staff that day were in fact agency staff. Nurses kept calling patients 'my sweet,' or 'darling' and the lady I was talking to posed the point as to whether this was a reason for why nurses are less respected these days. Whilst talking I recalled how the nursing sister on a ward where I once worked was formidable and woe betide should I ever call anyone anything different other than their name. Maybe it is down to these unidentified slips in relaxing the way we talk to each other that causes health care workers to receive less respect from the general public and allows patients to be so rude to the nursing staff as they are no longer seen as being professional due to the language they use. Reflecting back on when Hedge was on a children's ward, the nurses used to sit at the nurse's station with feet up on the desk, reclining back in their chairs whilst munching on sweets. I could never quite get my head around the fact that this was allowed. Or am I simply turning into a grumpy old lady! I hope not.

After chatting to the lady I went out to the foyer to get myself a drink and saw a patient in a bed being pushed by two porters who were more interested in their own conversation than engaging with the lady who was in her bed looking like a spare part. The lady on the bed raised her eyes at me and I smiled back. It is simple things like this that keeps me going as I know that I cannot give up the constant challenge of ensuring Hedge gets the care he needs.

My self-care on days like this is to wander down to the hospital shop and buy a sparkling water then attempt to climb the many flights of stairs back to the ward, reminding myself that this is meant to be good physical exercise (albeit not good for my joints).

However, by way of a reminder to myself from what a doctor once told me, pushing a wheelchair and assisting someone with their care adds to physical activity, so in a way I and many others like me are already squeezing in self-care when we don't even appreciate we are. However, approximately halfway up the stairwell I have to pretend that I am reading a message on my phone and pause in order to get my breath back. Little sis once said she would race me up the stairs; never again as I have told her it is dangerous to run up the stairs in case she knocks into anyone! Fortunately for me she thinks this is my true reason for not racing! Of course it is nothing to do with me being too unfit.

'THE UNOFFICIAL SELF-CARE GUIDE FOR CARERS'

Juggle the visits and appointments
Juggle the school runs too
Juggle the shopping, the laundry
Juggle the post and bills overdue

Juggle the housework and garden
Juggle the ordering of supplies
Juggle the changing of beds
Juggle the email replies

Juggle the fact that I work
Juggle the fact I am a wife
Juggle the fact I am a carer
Juggle the fact I have a life

Juggling is something I do
Juggling is how I survive
Juggling is learnt over time
Juggling keeps me alive

Juggling is part of self-care
Juggling needs to occur
Juggling enables time out
And gives gaps when days are a blur!

The spring of my winter

For the first time in a long time I felt like a weight was beginning to be lifted from my mind. I was listening to a well-known radio station today and a presenter was describing a new album and said it was like the spring to the artist's winter. The artist loved this description. I have to say that I love this phrase and it really does sum up days like today. How long this feeling will last for is unclear, but for now I feel lighter in mood and have a spring in my step.

Today was the day a new agency got all the new staff together for a staff induction at Hedge's house and much to my delight I was asked to talk about Hedge and what important issues the new team need to know. I was also able to show everyone in one go around the house, how to dismantle the mobility scooter etc. Usually this is done on a one-to-one basis, which takes up huge amounts of my time. However, today for the first time ever, a team has come together and really seem to want to make things happen for Hedge. His voice is not only being heard, but they have already been very strongly advocating for him on the ward.

Even better, Borry was rubbing noses with the kittens and didn't even growl at them when he came in for his food. This was a major milestone as old Borry was a very territorial cat and I was getting really stressed about his grumpy behaviour. I had read all the information and advice on attempting to introduce new kittens to an older male cat and was feeling like I had failed. I was so relieved that eventually the kittens were being accepted by my old boy. Best of all he even sauntered across to Hedge's house when I took the kittens there the other day and didn't seem to mind.

I was also invited out to a meal with a friend. I rarely go out for meals so I was really looking forward to this. Andrew had been away again and that also meant I had lost a few more pounds and he would have put some on. A tad mean I know, but it does make me feel better in myself knowing that I have lost a bit more weight than Andrew. I deliberated why it has been easier to lose weight this time, when on other occasions I have failed and I have realised that it is a combination of willpower and the fact that I have been so stressed that I have not really been feeling very hungry. I lost loads of weight after having Hedge and was very stressed then. So as an added bonus I have lost weight during a particularly stressful period of time whilst wrongly attributing it all as being down to my willpower. At least the scales are now good to stand on and even if stress has helped me on my way to a healthier weight then that must still be a good thing.

We were also very nearly closing in on the failings of the mental health team to address Hedge's needs. Although I knew in my heart of hearts that until it happened then we were still a long way off from receiving provision for Hedge. I could have done without a meeting with senior management on my extra special Birthday to discuss Hedge's needs again. Looking on the bright side, this did mean that Hedge's name was now known and people were recognising the failings.

Maybe just maybe I could relax enough to imagine for a moment that things might be looking up a bit. So alright maybe I did still have the outstanding concern regarding the Learning Disability Team and the formal complaint to do with the blocked catheter that was still unresolved, but things were progressing. Although a sloth could have the potential of moving quicker than some of the services who are meant to be supporting Hedge.

And last but not least I only had two thousand more words to write for this book. I have really enjoyed writing the book and yes this has also been time for self-care and I would strongly recommend writing down your own stories. My story is part of me and will be for many years to come after I am long dead and buried, figuratively speaking, but it is a story to tell and I am grateful for the fact that I have left something for others to learn about me and my family.

The spring to my winter
Could it really be?
A little bit of respite?
Some time for little me?

It may be a typical summer
Wet and cold again
But my little bit of spring
Is smiling through the rain

A new care team starting
Finally shifts complete
Hedge's support almost there
My batteries charged not deplete

My clothes fitting better
The house is still a mess
But I've done the garden
And managed to de-stress

The spring to my winter
It is so easy to see
New beginnings everywhere
And time for self-care for me

The storm after the calm

If I had anticipated that a slight lift in my spirits was to be long lived, then I was patently delusional. Less than two days after my happy dance, than things desperately deteriorated for Hedge. Somehow during the episode (that will no doubt haunt my dreams for many years) I was able to pull on my inner calm and keep a clear head. I will not describe the happenings that flashback into my memory, merely say that as a carer I have had many occasions when I think things cannot possibly get any harder and then they do. On leaving the hospital where Hedge was an inpatient I already had a sixth sense that I would be returning, so took the time to phone Andrew to explain to him that he would need to sort Little sis after I dropped her home from the childminder as I would have to return to the hospital. I returned to a state of affairs I had not really anticipated and ended up not getting home until the early hours of the morning. My whole body ached with the sheer exhaustion and my mind was in a fog. I somehow managed to drive home and update Andrew on the latest before falling into a vivid sleep.

I had to return to the hospital again before many cars were on the road and escaped just before midday. All the while my brain re-examining what had gone on and what had created the problem that I had somehow become part of. I imagine that many carers end up in this situation and probe the inner depths of their minds countless times on what they could have done to prevent complications from occurring. I am once again left mulling over what the future will bring and whether it will ever be to get Hedge home or whether he will end up living somewhere else instead.

In a way it is all very much 'closing the stable door after the horse has bolted' and even if Hedge did manage to get the mental health support he needed, five years is a long time to wait and there is so much more unpicking necessary. So in the afternoon after grabbing a coffee, Andrew motivated me and Little sis to go out for a drive and get fish and chips before coming home. Andrew intuitively knew I was exhausted and this gave me the lift I needed to carry on with the day.

I truly believe it is a balancing act to get the support you need. We now had a lovely care agency prepared to support Hedge but unless they received the training to deliver the support to Hedge then we might as well capitulate right then and there.

This is not the ending I wanted for the book, but sadly it is the ending in so many carers' lives that I have met. Thousands of carers like me are intolerably worn down and exhausted through the caring they provide. All the while services are ringfencing support and imposing restrictions for how you access the support.

I had a brief encounter with self-care by feeling selfish and going for a drive and then fish and chips. Tomorrow, who knows, but I do know that whatever the outcome I had done my utmost best to get Hedge the help he needs. For that moment in time I could rest knowing that I could have done no more to support him. If my efforts fail I will not be to blame for any negative outcomes due to Hedge's poor mental health. That has to be a good thing as I can then attempt self-care whilst truly being at peace with myself.

Finally taking stock of the situation

Having time to take stock and refocus life, I had successfully replanted the entire garden that was bereft of planting due to the years of building project work we were undertaking. The front garden was no longer a building site. My home was decluttered to the best of my ability. I wrote this book. I caught up with dental appointments and finally got in to school to discuss Little's sis and her needs. I commenced a parenting course and best of all lost nearly two stone in weight. I also learnt to stand my ground when the failing care agency once again tried to involve me in providing loads of care when they had more holes in cover than found in a Swiss cheese. I was also successful (almost) in helping Hedge see that whilst I remain on the end of the telephone, I am not at his every beck and call.

With regards to my work, I secured a job in a role that was right for me. I have been in my new job for just over a year and working additional hours most weeks on the staff bank and loving the combination of both my training role and clinical role.

The motorhome was sold, as it was only rubbing salt into our wounds about the lack of time we would ever get away in it. This was a huge decision for Andrew and me to make. It was a huge weight off our minds as the motorhome was no longer parked outside our house as a rather large reminder of the holidays we never had. Ridding ourselves of this rather large carbuncle also minimised our responsibilities and hassle of having to maintain it, insure it etc.

Andrew also successfully completed restoring the classic MGB Roadster that we had bought 25 years earlier at the start of our married life together.

And finally thank you Learning Disability Team (that I once worked for), for providing me with the opportunity to take stock and re-evaluate my life. I knew from the moment I was told that I had to increase my hours (when you knew this was impossible due to your refusal to validate Hedge to your service) that I would leave and move on to something better. I am enjoying pastures new, with absolutely no regrets, only sadness that a team who claim to be so supportive to people with learning disabilities are really not whom they pretend to be (apart from for the chosen few). I can now support Andrew whilst he is championing for Hedge as I will no longer have split allegiances. I can also challenge and expose the team's failings for Hedge and others without fear of being silenced. The best is that I can tell the world exactly how it is rather than having to be diplomatic because I work there. I no longer have to pretend I am someone I am not, I can be me with no frilly bits added on!

Taking stock
Not looking back
Planning ahead
And keeping track

Sorting through
The good and bad
Remembering
But never sad

Recapturing memories
An inward smile
Time to reflect
Just for a while

So much achieved
Some reflection too
Standing my ground
And keeping true

Hedge and Little sis
Now have a happier me
Re-energised and slimmer
Time to simply be

My enforced time out
Let me finally see
Life as it is
What I want for me

A work-life balance
Is needed by all
And self-care comes first
To avoid many a fall

Then there's my dream
One day care will be given
Not based on criteria
But needs-led driven

Then there was Covid -19

The start of 2020 was a strange time for most, for me it meant supporting the team I worked for with mask fit testing staff. At times it was just me and other times there was a group of us, testing one after another of a long queue of anxious colleagues. The smell of Bitrex, the substance used to test for the fit testing of the masks, clung to my clothes and skin and even showering once home did not get rid or dispel the bitter taste in my mouth. Day after day, hour after hour the same test, the same instructions, the same repetition. We were fortunate that the hospital where I work was extremely well prepared for the pandemic, but the whole environment was eerily strange. After the mask fit testing came the weeks of upskill training for staff and training for flexible support workers. The days became repetitive, déjà vu like, with each new group of staff being trained as though they were the first, lightening the mood, similar jokes, a smile of reassurance, a supportive nod. All whilst adhering to strict standards of hygiene – cleaning, re-cleaning and wiping of equipment.

On a plus side I also got to use the twisty garden twine that I had purchased many months before and used this to make the shape of a rainbow to hang on the tree outside my front door. Next I found a use for some of the thousands of plastic carrier bags stored in the kitchen. Little sis and me cut up coloured carrier bags into strips and tied them in colour order onto the twine shaped rainbow. I was and I still am proud of our achievement and at long last know that the years spent watching Blue Peter as a child had finally come into full use. I also got some self-care time whilst Little sis and myself sat down to make it.

Unfortunately, there was the added complication that Hedge was stuck in an interim placement as a direct result of lockdown and school had declined taking Little sis even though Andrew and myself were both key workers. Yes, life had become just a bit more complicated. Although complications can from time to time end up as a positive and for once my somewhat chaotic life was eased due to no school runs, no after school clubs, no packed lunches to make and finally no constant call outs by carers due to Hedge being in the interim placement. Actually life did become easier and I rather guiltily enjoyed lockdown: it was quicker to get to work, free parking at the hospital, no dash home to collect Little sis from school or the childminder. Maybe just maybe I was also feeling a tad smug about my life feeling better than it had been. However, I started to notice others really struggling as they had previously been afforded a more straightforward life that resembled nothing akin to the life me and other carers had been forced to live for years. I therefore wrote the following and posted it on some of the Facebook forums I belong to:

'This post is not meant to offend, but say it as it is. Life for me as a mother and unpaid carer to a disabled son has been pretty much been in lockdown since the day he was born. I was never able to do anything without huge logistic operations taking place, pre-planning and more often than not rescheduling or cancelling at the last moment. I have had some family members criticise me for not attending events or thinking I was making my son an excuse to not do things. I have been accused of bad parenting (you know who you are). I have spent many enforced days already in lockdown over the years caring for him in isolation in hospital cubicles or bays, where it was impossible to even get food to eat or sleep. Food would often perish if I bought too much. Shopping trips a luxury. I rarely had the opportunity to socialise, make friends and the friends I knew before having my son vanished. My world was very different to people I saw around me. I was forced to follow a lonely path to walk on, took a different view on life, and appreciated the small things in life that others took for granted. The chance to leave the house and even think about daily exercise never existed. My work as a nurse was my only escape. My passion to care and love for my work saw me through some very dark days. I never took time away from my work even when my son was seriously unwell in hospital as it was my chance to give to those who were in need. It was me time and allowed me a different life, often returning back to the ward to be with my son overnight.

I know that a lot of parents of disabled children with complex needs like my own son will be feeling things doubly bad as now their tiny chance of 'normality' to get out even for 5 minutes is no longer there. But like me you will have far more resilience than most, you have learnt to cope when others deserted you, you have learnt to pick yourself up and carry on going when smacked in the face with yet another unthinkable disaster. You can get through this new lockdown, as like me you have been there before, know how it feels and know that tomorrow will keep on coming only you will be stronger than before, because you know that being the parent of a child with disabilities you will never give in. You will cry tears, feel like screaming, but for once others are finally living some of the lonely life you have had to endure and maybe it may make the world a kinder place where people think more before they speak, actually mean it when they ask you how you are and no longer accuse you of poor parenting, as they are enduing some of what you have had to endure.

Someone in work asked me how my mental health was. Actually it is probably better than most right now as my life is really no different to what it has been for the last 20 years.

Keep strong, keep safe and be proud to already know what it feels like to be isolated. I know there are millions of carers out there, not just those of disabled children and like us they already know how it feels.'

The replies I had in response to this post were staggering with carers identifying with what I had written and saying how this post had made them feel not so alone. It appears I had hit the nail on the head for many. Maybe reading the same post here will also help others take a bit of something to help support self-care.

Wearing the dreaded face masks – keep smiling

Working on the Covid-19 escalation wards got me back to ward work again, but wearing the surgical masks and an apron has been and remains a challenge in hot weather. I have so far been one of the fortunate ones of not working whilst wearing full PPE (Personal Protective Equipment). I truly admire all those who do. However, when it was announced by the Prime Minister about the wearing of masks in the workplace I knew things were not looking that great and the fact that a lot of the offices in the hospital do not have any windows/good ventilation, it did not help with the feeling of claustrophobia for some. Wearing masks would now make it unbearable for not only hospital staff working directly with patients, but for everyone. I therefore wrote the following poem to lighten the mood. I honestly believe that a laugh can make all the difference and in this case there are so many plus points to mask wearing!

> To all those who despair
> And about to wear a mask

'THE UNOFFICIAL SELF-CARE GUIDE FOR CARERS'

Think of it as positive
As you go upon your task

Not only will you protect
Yourself and others too
But it'll help you calorie count
As upon your tongue you chew

'cause try as you might
It's hard to nibble all day
When a protective face mask
Is completely in the way

It also hides those wrinkles
And the odd hair upon your chin (for ladies of a certain age)
I forgot the dodgy teeth
It really is win win!

You can eat the spicy food at lunchtime
Your bad breath hidden away
Only you can smell it now
Not everyone along the way

And as for the best bit
Well I am really feeling smug
I almost look quite pretty
As I hide my ageing mug

Those passers-by might think
I'm like an English rose
Unaware of the obscure bits
Like lips in need of Botox and interesting nose

The list of positives just grows
For ladies just like me
My eyes are my best asset
And now it's all you see!

So I'll have a spring in my step
My COVID hairdo looking great
Almost looking like a young chick
Hiding my menopausal state

As for non-ageing females
Well the same applies to you
We can all imagine
You look amazing too

So to all those doubters
Who a mask they now must don
Think of all the plus points
And you won't go far wrong!

Covid-19 has affected everyone in the world differently, some have not come off too badly and others are grieving loss. For

Hedge it has delayed therapy once again, delayed care provision and prevented so much of his life from moving forwards. Yet more excuses piled onto other excuses. My brother was misdiagnosed when all the medical professionals wrongly assumed he had Covid-19 when it was in fact an infection that led to sepsis and resulted in a very long admission to hospital. Little sis is now totally disinterested in school due to having to self-entertain for the majority of the lockdown. Andrew is counting off the years to retirement. As for me it has been a different experience, almost heartening and hopefully it will make the world a kinder place for all to live in. I have learnt to sit back and enjoy the quiet, get on with my work and life as a mum without the constant nagging feeling that I should be packing more into my day (as I wasn't able to do this due to lockdown). I even got to enjoy my hair tied back as it was too long to keep down and rather enjoyed the mini facelift it gave me. There is always a plus side to life and self-care is always there; like me you just need a nudge sometimes to find it!

Lemons are great to suck on

From now on I will not be bothering to read happy posts of lovely looking people, bother looking up tasty food or hearing about children's wild achievements. Instead I shall be sucking on a lemon feeling frustrated that my life just doesn't quite match up to anyone else's and never will. I will plod on with greying hair and a face that looks more like that of a woman ten years older than me, remove all my mirrors so I don't have to look in them. I will sit in a dark cave pretending I am enjoying peace and quiet, whilst still chewing my lemon and ruminating 'why me?'. I will endeavour to join more forums where people are also having equally naff lives in order to give myself a boost and be grateful that my child is now a young adult and I don't have the next 20 years blissfully unaware of the hardship to come. If only they knew... Actually I already feel better as I do know about the hardship, I am already there, been there and done it, got the rhino skin, don't care what people think of me and how much their lives are better than mine. Alright so more accurately I do care, but am too tired to give a damn. All I can ask for is that when I finally meet the maker, that my child who has made me meet the maker early due to the stress he has given me, gives me a few years' peace before joining me. I am rather hoping that I am not alone in this view; otherwise I want to know your secret.

Keep smiling even if through gritted teeth. That's what helps me get though the day and believe me my front teeth are amazing due to having cost me a fortune as the result of Hedge accidentally knocking them out when his head smacked me in the mouth due to his low muscle tone. The dentist had only ever seen something like it before when he saw a jockey who had his teeth knocked out by a horse that had reared. Yep my gritted teeth look incredible and being positive about the whole experience I would never have had such good teeth if it had not been for Hedge. These great teeth allow me to suck on my lemon without any of the side effects of the lemon being too cold. It's got to be a win-win!!!

Remember there is always someone worse off and if you look in a mirror it is usually the reflection of yourself...

It's an age thing

I am now on the cusp of being 50 years old (there and beyond before this book is published and by the time it is being read). Where did that time go? In my mind I keep referring to how old my own parents were when I got married and how old I thought they were. Great, so I am now the same age.

So why is it that when you have a disabled child and have a younger body you have so much more help (admittedly with a battle) but then when you are completely run down from years of challenges and through sheer exhaustion, then the support network vanishes? Gone in the blink of a clock ticking from the 17th year to the 18th year.

I may be grey, have some wrinkles on my face, but I have life experience and enjoy nothing better than a good laugh and chat with my friends. My patience is less not because I am grumpy, but because I have been there dozens of times before and would really rather prefer not to keep repeating myself like a stuck record. I am weary and need a break from the constant stress and worry of having an adult child with complex needs and odd as it might or might not seem, I also need support and time for self-care.

When I get older
Attempting self-care
Will I get help any more?
Will I get the break I need?
Can I knock at your door?

When I get older
Motivation getting less
Will anyone help out?
Will anyone see me?
Or will I get exactly nowt?

When I get older
My patience growing tired
Will anyone care at all?
Will anyone bother to listen?
Or will I be taken as a fool?

A final update

It is bittersweet that after almost 21 years Hedge is still not receiving some of the services he should be. Hedge continues to be like Marmite, either loved or hated by those around him.

It is with great relief that I can announce that during Hedge's most recent admission the hospital's Learning Disability Team agreed to be involved as they recognised Hedge's need for their support based on the same report that the Community Learning Disability Team had turned down. The support received by the hospital's Learning Disability Team made a huge positive impact on the way Hedge's care was provided. The ward staff that cared for him were all supportive, kind and understanding. In the meantime, the Community Learning Disability Team is still refusing to acknowledge Hedge's needs due to them only providing support for the ringfenced few. The mental health support is still not forthcoming (this has been a need since 2014 and we are now in 2020). Hedge remains in an interim placement waiting for a package of care that can move forward with him living in his preferred place called home. Importantly, the staff from the care home remain supportive and strongly advocate Hedge's needs. Hedge's only Direct Payment carer continues to be employed to care for Hedge (thank goodness).

I continue to be working at the hospital in the Department of Professional Healthcare Education and also work clinical shifts at the local community hospital. Little sis remains a truly amazing Little sis to her big brother Hedge. As for Hedge, he proved his expressive writing skills by writing a really lovely Facebook thank you to the staff of the ward during his last admission to hospital (Hedge's receptive language skills remain a challenge). In the meantime, I continue emailing, telephoning, chasing and championing Hedge's needs in the hope that one day someone will listen and that he will receive care based on need, not due to convenience or based on funding.

Whilst all this is going on I will make sure I get a little piece of self-care each and every day as I am the story behind Hedge. I will take five, I will not feel guilty and I will never give in.

I bought a story book when Little sis was a toddler called 'The under the bed Monster'. The story was based on two possibilities and I see this fits well with my life so have rewritten this though the eyes of a carer to demonstrate how important self-care is.

A FINAL UPDATE

When a child is born there are two possibilities

Either the child is healthy or it is not

If the child is healthy that's that

Or if not the carer will start getting blamed

If the carer starts getting blamed there are two possibilities

Either the carer will shut up and go away and that's that

Or the carer will challenge and seek help and advice

If the carer challenges and seeks help and advice there are two possibilities

Either they will get fobbed off and that's that

Or they will refuse to listen and search out help

If they refuse to listen and search out help there are two possibilities

Either they will get exhausted and give in and that's that

Or they will continue to challenge

If they continue to challenge then there are two possibilities

Either they will finally get support they need and that's that

Or they will do it all themselves and lose all hope

If they do it all themselves and lose all
hope there are two possibilities

Either they will become tired and unwell and that's that

Or they will seek self-care and grow stronger in
caring for their child! (Whatever their child's age)

Acknowledgements

Andrew for his enduring patience.

Hedge and Little sis who inspire me daily to keep going.

Joanne for encouraging me to write yet
again and for sharing self-care.

Angie for the mutual telephone self-care time.

Carers past and present who love the 'Marmite' in Hedge.

Printed in Great Britain
by Amazon

54012042R00139